T0338482

IoT in Healthcare Systems

Implementing new information technologies into the healthcare sector can provide alternatives to managing patients' health records, systems, and improving the quality of care received. This book provides an overview of Internet of Things (IoT) technologies related to the healthcare field and covers the main advantages and disadvantages along with industry case studies.

This edited volume covers required standardization and interoperability initiatives, various Artificial Intelligence and Machine Learning algorithms, and discusses how health technology can meet the challenge of improving quality of life regardless of social and financial status, gender, age, and location. The book presents real-time applications and case studies in the fields of engineering, computer science, IoT, and healthcare and provides many examples of successful IoT projects.

The target audience for this edited volume includes researchers, practitioners, students, as well as key stakeholders involved in and working on healthcare engineering solutions.

Artificial Intelligence in Smart Healthcare Systems
Series Editors: Vishal Jain and Jyotir Moy Chatterjee

The progress of the healthcare sector is incremental as it learns from associations between data over time through the application of suitable big data and Internet of Things (IoT) frameworks and patterns. Many healthcare service providers are employing IoT-enabled devices for monitoring patient healthcare, but their diagnosis and prescriptions are instance-specific only. However, these IoT-enabled healthcare devices are generating volumes of data (Big-IoT Data) that can be analyzed for more accurate diagnosis and prescriptions. A major challenge in the above realm is the effective and accurate learning of unstructured clinical data through the application of precise algorithms. Incorrect input data leading to erroneous outputs with false positives shall be intolerable in healthcare as patients' lives are at stake. This new book series addresses various aspects of how smart healthcare can be used to detect and analyze diseases, the underlying methodologies, and related security concerns. Healthcare is a multidisciplinary field that involves a range of factors like the financial system, social factors, health technologies, and organizational structures that affect the healthcare provided to individuals, families, institutions, organizations, and populations. The goals of healthcare services include patient safety, timeliness, effectiveness, efficiency, and equity. Smart healthcare consists of m-health, e-health, electronic resource management, smart and intelligent home services, and medical devices. The IoT is a system comprising real-world things that interact and communicate with each other via networking technologies. The wide range of potential applications of IoT includes healthcare services. IoT-enabled healthcare technologies are suitable for remote health monitoring, including rehabilitation, assisted ambient living, etc. In turn, healthcare analytics can be applied to the data gathered from different areas to improve healthcare at a minimum expense.

This new book series is designed to be a first choice reference at university libraries, academic institutions, research and development centres, information technology centres, and any institutions interested in using, design, modelling, and analysing intelligent healthcare services. Successful application of deep learning frameworks to enable meaningful, cost-effective personalized healthcare services is the primary aim of the healthcare industry in the present scenario. However, realizing this goal requires effective understanding, application, and amalgamation of IoT, big data, and several other computing technologies to deploy such systems in an effective manner. This series shall help clarify the understanding of certain key mechanisms and technologies helpful in realizing such systems.

Designing Intelligent Healthcare Systems, Products, and Services Using Disruptive Technologies and Health Informatics
Teena Bagga, Kamal Upreti, Nishant Kumar, Amirul Hasan Ansari, and Danish Nadeem

Next Generation Healthcare Systems Using Soft Computing Techniques
D. Rekh Ram Janghel, Rohit Raja, and Korhan Cengiz

IoT In Healthcare Systems

Applications, Benefits, Challenges, and Case Studies

Edited by
Piyush Kumar Shukla, Aditya Patel,
Prashant Kumar Shukla, Prashant Parashar,
and Basant Tiwari

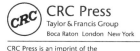

CRC Press
Taylor & Francis Group
Boca Raton London New York

CRC Press is an imprint of the
Taylor & Francis Group, an **informa** business

Designed cover image: © Shutterstock

First edition published 2023
by CRC Press
6000 Broken Sound Parkway NW, Suite 300, Boca Raton, FL 33487-2742

and by CRC Press
4 Park Square, Milton Park, Abingdon, Oxon, OX14 4RN

CRC Press is an imprint of Taylor & Francis Group, LLC

© 2023 Taylor & Francis Group, LLC

Library of Congress Cataloging-in-Publication Data
Names: Shukla, Piyush Kumar, 1976– editor. | Patel, Aditya, editor. |
Shukla, Prashant Kumar, editor.
Title: IoT in healthcare systems : applications, benefits, challenges and case studies /
edited by Piyush Kumar Shukla, Aditya Patel and Prashant Kumar Shukla.
Description: First edition. | Boca Raton : CRC Press, 2023. |
Series: Artificial intelligence in smart healthcare systems |
Includes bibliographical references and index.
Identifiers: LCCN 2022047379 | ISBN 9780367702144 (hardback) |
ISBN 9780367702151 (paperback) | ISBN 9781003145035 (ebook)
Subjects: LCSH: Internet of things. | Internet in medicine. |
Medical informatics–Technological innovations. |
Artificial intelligence–Medical applications.
Classification: LCC RC859.7.I58 I58 2023 |
DDC 610.285/63–dc23/eng/20230202
LC record available at https://lccn.loc.gov/2022047379

ISBN: 978-0-367-70214-4 (hbk)
ISBN: 978-0-367-70215-1 (pbk)
ISBN: 978-1-003-14503-5 (ebk)

DOI: 10.1201/9781003145035

Typeset in Times
by Newgen Publishing UK

Contents

About the Editors

Piyush Kumar Shukla is Associate Professor in the Department of Computer Science and Engineering at the University Institute of Technology, Rajiv Gandhi Proudyogiki Vishwavidyalaya (Technological University of Madhya Pradesh), India. He has 15 years of experience in teaching and research. He completed a Post Doctorate Fellowship under the Information Security Education and Awareness Project Phase II funded by the Ministry of Electronics and Information Technology, SVNIT Surat, India. His research interests include white-box cryptography, information security and privacy, cyber security, dynamic wireless networks, machine learning, the Internet of Things, image processing, and Blockchain. In addition to publishing more than 15 Indian patents and around 10 papers in international journals, he was awarded Best Researcher of the Year 2019 for Outstanding Research Contribution. Shukla is a senior life member of the IEEE.

Aditya Patel is Assistant Professor in the Department of Computer Science and Engineering, Lakshmi Narain College of Technology Bhopal. He has worked on more than 50 websites and software and has four years of teaching experience in various reputed technical colleges and universities along with two years of industry experience. His current research areas are machine learning, deep learning, and the Internet of Things.

Prashant Kumar Shukla is Assistant Professor and Research Coordinator in Jagran Lakecity University, India. His research interests include machine learning, deep learning, computer vision, the Internet of Things, software engineering, computer networking, mobile computing, information security, Python, and Java programming. He has 13 patents and has published and presented more than 17 research papers in various national and international journals and conferences. He received the Innovative Teacher award from GISR Foundation and the American College of Dubai. He also was awarded Best Researcher by ESN Publications. He is also associated with two start-ups.

Prashant Parashar is an experienced information security professional with around 16 years of experience in the information security domain. He is Security Analyst at Betfair, UK. His experience includes Align IT security governance, information security management, auditing and compliance, information security metrics, development and implementation of information security policy, and procedures and ISMS implementation in line with ISO 27001 requirements.

Basant Tiwari is Assistant Professor in the Computer Science and Engineering Department at Hawassa University, Ethiopia. His area of research is pervasive computing in healthcare and the Internet of Things and information and network security. He is a senior member of IEEE, a senior member of ACM, and a life member of CSI and IACSIT. He also chairs at iMPLab situated at Bhopal, India. Tiwari has organized various national and international conferences, delivered talks, and chaired technical sessions.

1 Artificial Intelligence-Based Smart Medical Services

Dhanasekaran Arumugam,[1]
Christopher Stephen,[2] Vishnupriyan Jegadeesan,[1]
Ajay John Paul,[3] Arunpillai Viswanathan Harish,[1]
Krishna S.,[1] and Gunalan K.[1]
[1] Chennai Institute of Technology, Madras, India
[2] Dr. Sagunthala R&D Institute of Science and Technology, Chennai, India
[3] Kyungpook National University, Daegu, South Korea

CONTENTS

DOI: 10.1201/9781003145035-1

1

1.1   INTRODUCTION

A healthcare system allows patients and doctors to communicate with each other and remotely exchange information that is monitored, collected, and analysed from patients' daily activities via the Internet of Things. Smart healthcare is defined as the integration of patients and doctors onto a common platform for intelligent health monitoring through the analysis of daily human activities [1].

Due to the massive rise in population, traditional healthcare is unable to meet everyone's demands. Medical services are not accessible or expensive despite having excellent infrastructure and cutting-edge technologies [2]. Further, in healthcare service delivery, resource shortages and uneven allocation can put additional strain on already overburdened providers. Smart healthcare is emerging as a critical strategy for addressing these issues and personalizing healthcare.

The main objective of smart healthcare is to assist consumers by informing them about their medical conditions and keeping them informed about their health. Smart healthcare allows people to handle various emergency circumstances on their own. It focuses on increasing the user's quality of life and experience. Smart healthcare is the integration of disparate healthcare delivery mechanisms; it employs electronic patient records and streamlines processes with the goal of improving people's lives by lowering health risks and increasing well-being. Patient-centric services, such as remote monitoring and checks, can be tailored to the patient's specific requirements and have a broader reach, improving access to healthcare. Because of the ageing population's increased life expectancy and the rise in chronic diseases, effective remote monitoring of health conditions and the adoption of smart healthcare products are gaining traction [3].

Smart healthcare enables the most efficient use of available resources, remote patient monitoring, lowers the cost of treatment for the user, and enables the medical professionals to expand their services across geographical barriers. With the growing trend toward smart cities, an effective smart healthcare system ensures that its residents live a healthy lifestyle. In general, connected health refers to any digital healthcare solution that can operate remotely, and it is a catch-all term for subsets like telemedicine and mobile-health, but with the addition of continuous health monitoring, emergency detection, and automatically alerting appropriate individuals.

The objective of connected health is to improve the quality and efficiency of healthcare by allowing self-care and supplementing it with remote care. Its roots can be traced back to the telemedicine era, when users were educated about their health and given feedback as needed. Smart healthcare refers to solutions that can run totally on their own, whereas connected healthcare refers to systems that allow consumers to receive feedback from clinicians. Figure 1.1 shows a typical framework of a smart healthcare system.

To maintain consistent internet connectivity and sustain large data traffic in a hospital setting where a healthcare network is maintained, Wi-Fi and ground cables are essential. On-body sensors and stationary medical devices are two types of medical equipment used to achieve smart healthcare. Biosensors that are attached to the human body for physiological monitoring are known as on-body sensors. In-vitro

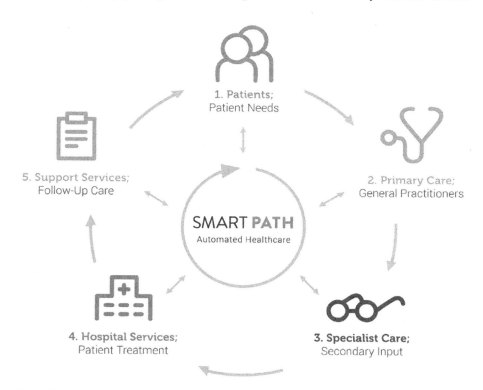

FIGURE 1.1 Typical framework of smart healthcare system [4].

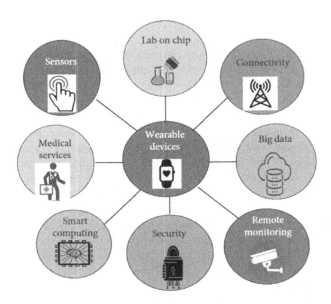

FIGURE 1.2 Components of a smart healthcare system.

and in-vivo sensors are two different types of sensors. In-vitro sensors are externally attached to the human body, decreasing the need for lab or hospital facilities in healthcare. In-vivo sensors are implantable devices that are inserted inside the body after meeting all sterilizing regulations and standards. Figure 1.2 depicts the four major components of healthcare systems: identification, location, sensing, and connectivity. Emergency services, smart computing, sensors, remote monitoring, wearable devices, connectivity devices, and big data are all used to implement smart healthcare [5].

1.2 CLASSIFICATION OF SMART HEALTHCARE

Smart healthcare can be divided into functional requirements and non-functional requirements as shown in Figure 1.3. Functional requirements address specific criteria, such as the range of operation of the thermistor/thermometer, data collection method, and frequency of operation of a temperature monitoring system. Hence, functional requirements vary depending on the application of each component in the healthcare system. Non-functional requirements are characteristics that can be used to assess the quality of a healthcare system and can be further divided into performance criteria and ethical requirements. Performance criteria can be further split into software and hardware requirements [6].

The criteria for an efficient smart healthcare system are lower power, small form factor, reliability, quality in service, enriched user experience, higher efficiency, ability to interoperate across different platforms, ease of deployment, scalability of the system to upgrade to newer versions and technologies, and ample connectivity.

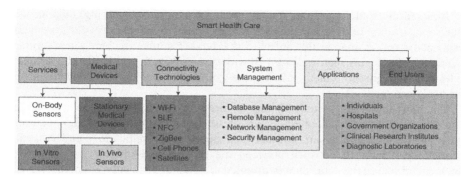

FIGURE 1.3   Classification of smart healthcare.

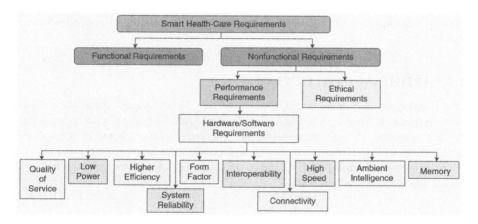

FIGURE 1.4   The requirements in smart healthcare.

The requirements of smart healthcare are shown in Figure 1.4.

Sensors or actuators, computing devices, data-storage elements, and networking components can be used to categorise smart healthcare system components. A sensor is an analytical device and when it combines with a biological element it produces a signal for recognition of events [7]. Sensors and actuators differ depending on the monitoring system. The most common sensors used in smart healthcare are temperature sensors, electrocardiogram (ECG), blood pressure, blood glucose, electromyogram, heart rate, oxygen saturation, gyroscope, motion sensors, and accelerometers. Computing devices range from smartphones, tablets, and personal digital assistants to complex and advanced devices such as supercomputers and servers. Memory is crucial in smart healthcare because storing information is the most important function of these systems. The data-storage components in the smart healthcare network span a broader spectrum, including embedded memory on sensing devices and large servers used for big-data analytics.

Link sensors, routers, and base stations are all examples of networking components. The sophistication of the components varies according to the severity of the problem being addressed. A smart healthcare network is built on wireless technologies. Various wireless technologies such as Wi-Fi, Bluetooth, 6LoWPAN, and RFID play critical roles in exchanging information among the various physical elements that comprise the healthcare network.

The most important system designs required for a smart healthcare system are app oriented, things oriented, and semantics oriented. App-oriented architectures must ensure reliable transmission between smartphone applications and sensors, create a personalised network between the sensors and the user's computing device, and secure the data. Things-oriented architectures must be adaptable based on the application, provide real-time monitoring, on-time delivery, greater sensitivity, maintain higher efficiency at lower power dissipation, and engage in intelligent processing. Semantic-oriented systems should be able to develop behavioural patterns based on previously acquired information, use natural-language processing techniques to improve user experience, and be capable of ubiquitous computing. [8].

1.3 ARTIFICIAL INTELLIGENCE

The simulation of human intelligence processes by machines, particularly computer systems, is known as Artificial Intelligence (AI). Expert systems, natural language processing, speech recognition, and machine vision are some of the specific applications of AI. Humans are being replaced by machines, robots, and similar innovations with the use of AI. AI uses a huge amount of data to process a task and makes accurate and desired results.

1.3.1 PROCESS OF AI

AI programming focuses on three cognitive skills: learning, reasoning, and self-correction.

1.3.1.1 Learning Processes

Learning process focuses on acquiring data and creating rules to create the data into actionable information. The rules, which are named as algorithms, provide computing devices with step-by-step instructions to complete a specific task.

1.3.1.2 Reasoning Processes

Reasoning process focuses on selecting the right algorithm to obtain a desired outcome.

1.3.1.3 Self-Correction Processes

Self-correction processes are designed to continually refine the algorithms to enable to provide the most accurate outcome [9]. The process of AI is shown in Figure 1.5.

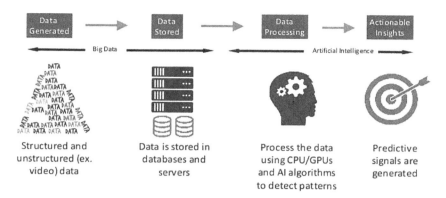

FIGURE 1.5 The process of AI.

1.3.2 TYPES OF AI

AI is often classified in the following categories:

- Reactive AI, which relies on real-time data to make decisions.
- Limited Memory AI, which relies on stored data to make decisions.
- Theory of Mind AI, which considers subjective elements such as user intent when making decisions.
- Self-Aware AI, which possesses a human-like consciousness that is capable of independently setting goals and using data to decide the best way to achieve an objective.

The basic components of any AI are learning, reasoning, problem solving, perception, and using language. Figure 1.6 shows some of the components of typical AI [10].

1.4 THE HEALTHCARE INDUSTRY

The world today is driven by data. Data has become essential in all sectors of the economy, such as in consumer goods, real estate, healthcare, manufacturing, or any other industry. With more and more applications of data, the world is moving towards or to be more precise undergoing the biggest economic and technological transformations of all time. The healthcare industry is huge and is made up of the following elements.

1.4.1 THE ELEMENTS OF HEALTHCARE INDUSTRIES

1.4.1.1 Hospitals and Clinics

Hospitals and clinics are the infrastructural components of any healthcare industry that act as a starting point for all kinds of medical needs. They recommend a certain number of tests and medicines, which are paving towards all the other elements of the healthcare industry. People who are frequent hospital visitors or are health-oriented are also driven towards the medical insurance industry.

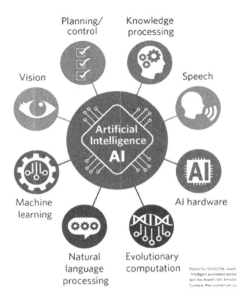

FIGURE 1.6   Components of typical AI.

1.4.1.2   The Pharmaceutical Industries

The pharmaceutical industries are one of the most important elements of the healthcare industry. They produce drugs and medicines and decide a price point of the drug depending on various factors like demand, rarity, etc.

1.4.1.3   The Medical Insurance Agencies

The human body is always exposed to medical uncertainties. The fear of spending more when a crisis creeps in acts as a bait for these companies to bring in customers. Individuals invest in medical insurances by paying a premium amount in installments and hence saving a huge amount when a medical emergency kicks in. Today private companies also provide medical insurances to their employees and family members, which drives huge revenues for companies working in the medical insurance domain.

1.4.1.4   Pathology and Lab Tests

The medical test market is huge. From blood tests to large CT scans, people visit these labs and get their tests done regularly, which makes it a need of the hour. Most people get their tests done to keep up with their general well-being. Thus, these labs are an important element of the healthcare industry.

1.4.2   THE NEED FOR AI IN THE HEALTHCARE INDUSTRY

AI is the cutting-edge technology of all the economic sectors. The healthcare industry is one of the major sections of the economy and is growing swiftly. This growth translates to more people concerned about their health, which translates into more people participating in the healthcare chain (i.e., going to the hospital and ending up spending money on the associated costs).

Due to the more and more people being involved in the digital platform, more and more data are coming into the picture and with the huge involvement of data, AI is being used for doing things better and. The application of AI has proved to be a kind of symbiotic for both the parties – the ones who are driving it and the ones who are availing the benefits of it.

The healthcare industry forms almost 12% of any developed or developing country's economy by making the best use of the resources available with it, which are nothing but stored in the form of data. The health data of billions are stored in the form of hospital records, medical prescriptions, pathology reports, etc. AI makes the best use of this data, and is driving the healthcare industry in the following ways.

1.4.2.1 Optimizing Cost Plans and Structures

With the huge amount of data available, hospitals can plan better on when to spend and when to curtail. Also, these units can analyze the consumer needs and charge accordingly. With big data, analysis of various costs and formulating strategies for better functioning of these medical units has become easy. With the growing number of people, economies of scale can be achieved and the benefits of it can be delivered to the ones seeking services and also to the ones who are driving such plans with the help of huge data present with them.

1.4.2.2 Supply Chain Efficiencies for Pharmaceutical Companies

With the availability of the huge amount of clinical and patient data drug manufacturers can easily analyze the medical conditions and histories for a certain group of individuals and the medicines they use regularly. With AI, these companies segregate zones based on geopolitical boundaries, medical similarities, disease rarity, etc., and devise methods to deliver their medicines based on such parameters. Also, with the help of the data they use AI to finalize price points of various drugs based on diseases that can be cured. The pharma sector is making the best possible use of AI, which in turn is making medicines accessible to patients and also helping pharmaceutical companies expand their market shares.

1.4.2.3 Healthcare Insurance Market

With the availability of patient data based on the medical conditions, a well-curated insurance plan can be chalked out and presented. The medical insurance market has a huge database of people, their medical conditions, details of their family members, etc., which gives them an edge and AI makes the best use of this available data.

1.4.2.4 The Fitness Industry

The fitness industry is a multi-billion-dollar industry. People keep tabs on their health and well-being all the time. Applications like Google Fit are installed on phones and these apps track fitness-related information, generating a huge amount of data every second. These data can be both generic and individual specific. Corporations track consumer needs through these kinds of applications and then use these insights for providing tailor-made solutions and hence making money. With the help of AI, the healthcare industry is operating digitally and successfully.

1.4.2.5 The Government

The government makes use of this health data to develop various schemes. With the help of AI, the government can also track the performance of the healthcare industry, which translates into an economic indicator of growth and progress. The government also uses this huge amount of data to keep a constant tab on the number of hospitals in a particular area, the medical supplies needed on a regular basis, availability of doctors and nurses in a particular area, outbreak of various calamities and communicable diseases, eradication of serious diseases like polio, malaria, dengue, etc. With the help of this data, the government educates a lot of people and helps them in the upkeep of their well-being.

With AI coming into play, the healthcare industry has drastically evolved. The whole industry has been taken away by the wave of digitization and companies aiming to track information and bring in data points every minute. Real-time information can be tracked with the help of AI. Hospitals are getting more efficient, planning out their staff better, becoming more available for people so that they can reap the best possible outcomes.

Pharma companies can generate huge revenues by supplying medicines to countries where there is demand and hence channelizing their supplies and revenue streams. The insurance market is becoming bigger and better. The availability of data is being translated into sales and revenues every hour. The healthcare industry and the amount of data involved in this industry surprised the whole world. Also, the money involved in such industry for data and AI is insane. Will AI prove to be a boon or a bane is the debate of the future but right now it is making the world fast and the health space small and close [11].

1.5   APPLICATIONS OF AI IN MEDICINE TODAY

1.5.1   DIAGNOSE DISEASES

In order to correctly diagnose illnesses years of medical training is required. The diagnostics processes are lengthy and time-consuming, which puts doctors under a lot of pressure, and it frequently causes life-saving patient diagnoses to be delayed. Machine Learning, particularly deep learning algorithms, have recently made huge advances in automatically diagnosing diseases, making diagnostics cheaper and more accessible.

Machine Learning algorithms can learn to recognise patterns in the same way as doctors do. But, the algorithms involved in ML require a large number of actual instances and therefore, the information should be digitized for accurate results. Machine Learning is particularly helpful in areas where the diagnostic information a doctor examines is already digitized such as:

- CT scans can be used to detect lung cancer or strokes.
- Using electrocardiograms and cardiac MRI scans to assess the risk of sudden cardiac death or other heart disorders.

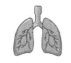

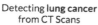

Detecting **lung cancer** from CT Scans   Assess **cardiac health** from electrocardiograms   Classify **skin lesions** from images of the skin   Identify **retinopathy** from eye images

FIGURE 1.7 Diagnostic information flow using AI.

- Classifying skin lesions in skin images.
- Finding indicators of diabetic retinopathy in eye images.

Figure 1.7 illustrates the diagnostic information flow of AI.

Algorithms are becoming as proficient as experts at diagnosing since there is so much quality data available in many situations. The algorithm may provide findings in a fraction of a second and can be simply be copied anywhere. Furthermore ambitious systems involve the combination of multiple data sources such as CT, MRI, genomics and proteomics, patient data, and even handwritten files, for providing an opinion about a disease or its progression. The AI technologies will alert experts to potentially cancerous tumours or risky cardiac rhythms, allowing doctors to concentrate on the interpretation of such signals.

1.5.2 FASTER DRUG DEVELOPMENT

Drug development is a costly procedure. AI can improve the efficiency of many of the analytical techniques used in drug development that can save time and cost involved in the drug development process. AI has already been used successfully in all the main stages of drug development such as identifying targets for intervention, discovering drug candidates, speeding up clinical trials, and finding biomarkers for diagnosing the disease, discussed as follows.

1.5.2.1 Identify Targets for Intervention

Understanding the basic origins of a disease as well as its resistance mechanisms is the first step in therapeutic development. Then the determination of targets is used to treat the condition. The growing availability of high-throughput tools like shRNA screening and deep sequencing has considerably enhanced the quantity of data accessible for identifying suitable target pathways. Traditional methods, on the other hand, still struggle to integrate the large number and variety of data sources – and then uncover the appropriate patterns. Machine Learning algorithms can more easily analyse all the available data and can even learn to automatically identify good target proteins. Figure 1.8 shows different stages of drug development.

1.5.2.2 Discover Drug Candidates

Identifying a compound that can interact with the identified target molecule in the desired way is the second stage in drug development, and involves screening a large

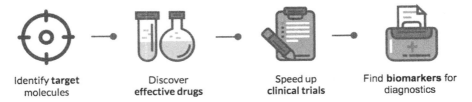

Identify **target**   Discover   Speed up   Find **biomarkers** for
molecules   **effective drugs**   **clinical trials**   diagnostics

FIGURE 1.8   Different stages of drug development.

number of potential compounds for their effect on the target, not to mention their off-target side effects. These compounds can be natural, synthetic, or bioengineered. However, current software is often inaccurate and produces a lot of bad suggestions. Thus, it takes a very long time to narrow down the best drug candidates. AI algorithms can also assist in this area, since they can learn to anticipate a molecule's compatibility based on structural fingerprints and chemical descriptors and then sift through millions of possible molecules narrowing down the best alternatives (i.e., those with the fewest adverse effects). Thus, saving a lot of time in medication development.

1.5.2.3   Speed Up Clinical Trials

It is very difficult to find suitable candidates for clinical trials. If the wrong candidates are selected, it will prolong the trial costing a lot of time and resources. Machine Learning algorithms can help speed up the design of clinical trials by automatically selecting acceptable candidates and ensuring that groups of trial participants are distributed correctly. Algorithms can aid in the detection of patterns that distinguish quality candidates. Moreover, they can also act as an early warning system for clinical trials that are not yielding solid findings, thus allowing researchers to intervene sooner and save the drug's development.

1.5.2.4   Find Biomarkers for Diagnosing the Disease

Better treatment can be possible only if they are thoroughly understood. Whole genome sequencing is exceedingly costly and requires specialised lab equipment as well as professional knowledge. Biomarkers are chemicals that are present in biological fluids that can determine whether or not a patient has a disease with 100% certainty. They make identifying an illness both safe and affordable and also provide data that can be used to pinpoint the progression of the disease. Thus, making it easier for doctors to choose the correct treatment and monitor whether the drug is working.

However, discovering suitable biomarkers for a particular disease is a hard, expensive, and time-consuming process that involves screening tens of thousands of potential molecule candidates. AI can speed up the process by automating a major percentage of the manual effort. The algorithms divide molecules into excellent and bad candidates, allowing physicians to focus on the most promising options. Biomarkers can be used to identify:

- The presence of a disease as early as possible – diagnostic biomarker
- The risk of a patient developing the disease – risk biomarker

- The likely progress of a disease – prognostic biomarker
- Whether a patient will respond to a drug – predictive biomarker

1.5.3 PERSONALIZE TREATMENT

Diverse patients have different reactions to medications and therapy regimens. As a result, tailored therapy has huge potential to extend patients' lives. However, determining the characteristics that influence therapy selection is difficult. Machine Learning can help to determine the variables to suggest that a patient will have a certain reaction to a given treatment by automating this complex statistical work. As a result, the algorithm can forecast a patient's likely reaction to a given therapy. The system learns this by cross-referencing similar patients and comparing their treatments and outcomes. The resulting outcome predictions make it much easier for doctors to design the right treatment plan.

1.5.4 IMPROVE GENE EDITING

Clustered Regularly Interspaced Short Palindromic Repeats (CRISPR), specifically the CRISPR-Cas9 system for gene editing, is a big leap forward toward editing DNA cost effectively and precisely, like a surgeon. Short guide RNAs (sgRNA) can be used in this approach to target and edit a specific place on the DNA. However, the guide RNA can suit several DNA sites, which might result in unexpected consequences. A key bottleneck in the use of the CRISPR technology is the careful selection of guide RNA with the fewest hazardous side effects. When it comes to forecasting the degree of both guide-target interactions and off-target effects for a particular sgRNA, machine learning models have been shown to yield the best outcomes. This might hasten the synthesis of guide RNA for every segment of human DNA [12].

1.6 CLINICAL APPLICATIONS

Improvements in computing power resulting in faster data collection and data processing, growth of genomic sequencing databases, widespread implementation of electronic health record systems, and improvements in natural language processing and computer vision, enabling machines to replicate human perceptual processes, have all occurred during this half-century period, enabling the growth of healthcare-related applications of AI. Some of the clinical applications of AI are as follows.

1.6.1 CARDIOVASCULAR

AI algorithms have demonstrated promising results in accurately diagnosing and risk stratifying patients with coronary artery disease, indicating their utility as an initial triage tool [13, 14] despite the fact that few studies have directly compared machine learning model accuracy to clinician diagnostic ability [15].

Other algorithms have been used to predict patient mortality, medication effects, and adverse events after acute coronary syndrome treatment. Internet-based technologies have also demonstrated the ability to monitor patients' cardiac data points, increasing the amount of data and the various settings AI models can use and potentially enabling earlier detection of cardiac events that occur outside of the hospital [16].

Another area of growing interest is the use of AI in classifying heart sounds and diagnosing valvular disease [17].

The limited data available to train machine learning models, such as limited data on social determinants of health as they relate to cardiovascular disease, has been one of the challenges of AI in cardiovascular medicine [18].

1.6.2 AI APPLICATION IN STROKE

The occurrence of a stroke, which affects over 500 million individuals worldwide, is a very common and frequently seen disease. In Middle Asia, it is the leading cause of death, while in North America, it is one of the leading causes. As a result, research into stroke prevention and treatment is extremely beneficial. AI techniques can assist in three fundamental categories of stroke care:

- Predicting a stroke and detecting it in advance
- Treating it if diagnosed
- Prediction of outcomes and assessment of prognosis

1.6.2.1 Early Diagnosis

When blood flow to the brain is poor, cells die, resulting in a stroke, which is frequently triggered by thrombus build-up in vessels, hence the term cerebral infarction. Many patients have been unable to receive timely treatment due to late recognition of stroke symptoms. Villar et al. created a device that detects movement and predicts the onset of a stroke. It is based on the principles of two well-known Machine Learning algorithms: PCA (principal component analysis) and genetic fuzzy finite state machine. The recognition of movement patterns is used in the detecting procedure. When movement patterns deviate from normal, it signals a stroke warning that should be investigated as soon as feasible. For disease evaluation, such as in the case of stroke diagnosis, neuroimaging procedures such as CT scan and MRI are required. Machine Learning approaches have been used by researchers to analyse neuroimaging data. When applied to a CT scan, Machine Learning methods aid in the detection of free-floating intraluminal thrombus in carotid plaque. To keep track of the possibilities of strokes, Rehme et al. used a well-known Machine Learning programme called support vector machine, or SVM. In this situation, SVM had an accuracy rate of roughly 87%. Griffs et al. used Bayes classification in the stroke identification method. The computer-assisted method produced results that were extremely similar to those obtained by human specialists. In multimodal brain MRI, Kamnitsas et al. used 3D CNN for lesion segmentation. Rondina et al. performed the Gaussian method regression on few sample MRI data to find a convincing result of predicted features.

1.6.2.2 Treatment

The visualisation and survival rate are linked to the result of intravenous thrombolysis as a serious activity of crisis measurement. Patients receiving tPA treatment by CT scan were studied to see if they experienced symptomatic cerebral bleeding. Whole-brain scans were used as input for SVM, and the results beat traditional radiology-based approaches. Predicting the outcome and determining the prognosis Multiple factors influence stroke prognosis and illness mortality. When compared to traditional methods, machine learning algorithms have shown to be more accurate. Zhang et al. created a model to support the process of clinical decision-making by utilising logistic regression and analysing physiological indicators for a time period of 48 hours following the incidence of stroke in order to predict the outcome of three-month period. Asadi and colleagues compiled a database that included 107 patients who had intra-arterial therapy for acute posterior or anterior circulation stroke. The authors used SVM and a simulated neural system to analyse the data and attained a precision of over 70%. They also employed machine learning to identify characteristics that influence the outcome of brain arteriovenous contortion, which may be treated with endovascular embolization. A standard regression inquiry model could only get a precision ratio of 43 percent, but their tactics performed admirably with a precision of 97.5 percent [19].

1.6.3 DERMATOLOGY

Dermatology is an imaging-rich specialty, and the evolution of deep learning has been closely linked to image processing. As a result, dermatology and deep learning are a natural fit [20]. In dermatology, there are three types of imaging: contextual images, macro images, and micro images. Deep learning demonstrated significant progress in each modality [21]. Han et al. showed keratinocytic skin cancer detection from face photographs [22]. Esteva et al. demonstrated dermatologist-level classification of skin cancer from lesion images [23], Noyan et al. demonstrated a convolutional neural network that achieved 94% accuracy at identifying skin cells from microscopic Tzanck smear images [24]. Recent advances have suggested that artificial intelligence (AI) could be used to describe and evaluate the outcome of maxillo-facial surgery or the assessment of cleft palate therapy in terms of facial attractiveness or age appearance [25,26] An artificial intelligence system can detect skin cancer more accurately. Human dermatologists correctly identified 86.6% of skin cancers from images, compared to 95% for the CNN machine [27].

1.6.4 GASTROENTEROLOGY

AI has the potential to play a role in many aspects of gastroenterology. Endoscopic procedures such as esophagogastroduodenoscopies (EGD) and colonoscopies rely on the detection of abnormal tissue in a short period of time. By incorporating AI into these endoscopic procedures, clinicians can more quickly identify diseases, assess their severity, and visualise blind spots. Early trials of AI detection systems for early gastric cancer revealed sensitivity comparable to that of expert endoscopists [28].

1.6.5 INFECTIOUS DISEASES

AI has demonstrated promise in both the laboratory and clinical settings of infectious disease medicine. As the novel coronavirus wreaks havoc around the world, the United States is expected to invest more than $2 billion in AI-related healthcare research by 2025, more than four times what was spent in 2019. Neural networks have been developed to detect a host response to COVID 19 from mass spectrometry samples in a timely and accurate manner [29]. Other applications include antimicrobial resistance detection using support vector machines, machine learning analysis of blood smears to detect malaria, and improved point-of-care Lyme disease testing based on antigen detection. AI has also been studied for improving meningitis, sepsis, and tuberculosis diagnosis, as well as predicting treatment complications in hepatitis B and hepatitis C patients [30].

1.6.6 ONCOLOGY

AI has been studied for its potential applications in cancer diagnosis, risk stratification, tumour molecular characterization, and cancer drug discovery. The ability to accurately predict which treatment protocols will be best suited for each patient based on their individual genetic, molecular, and tumor-based characteristics is a particular challenge in oncologic care that AI is being developed to address [31]. AI has been trialled in cancer diagnostics with the reading of imaging studies and pathology slides due to its ability to translate images to mathematical sequences [32]. In January 2020, researchers demonstrated an AI system based on a Google DeepMind algorithm that outperformed human breast cancer detection experts [33,34]. It was reported in July 2020 that an AI algorithm developed by the University of Pittsburgh achieves the highest accuracy in identifying prostate cancer to date, with 98 percent sensitivity and 97 percent specificity [35,36].

1.6.7 PATHOLOGY

Pathological analysis of cells and tissues is widely regarded as the gold standard for disease diagnosis in many cases. Artificial intelligence-assisted pathology tools have been developed to aid in the diagnosis of a variety of diseases, including hepatitis B, gastric cancer, and colorectal cancer. AI has also been used to forecast genetic mutations and disease outcomes. [37]. AI is well-suited for use in low-complexity pathological analysis of large-scale screening samples, such as colorectal or breast cancer screening, alleviating pathologists' workload and allowing for faster sample analysis turnaround [38]. Several deep learning and artificial neural network models have demonstrated accuracy comparable to that of human pathologists, and a study of deep learning assistance in diagnosing metastatic breast cancer in lymph nodes revealed that the accuracy of humans with the assistance of a deep learning programme was higher than that of humans alone or the AI programme alone [39]. The implementation of digital pathology is expected to save a university centre more than $12 million over the course of five years, though the savings attributed to AI specifically have not yet been widely researched [40]. Since the areas of concern can be highlighted on a pathology sample and present them in real-time to a pathologist for more efficient review, augmented and virtual reality could be a stepping stone to wider implementation of AI-assisted pathology. The lack of prospective, randomised, multi-center-controlled trials in determining the true clinical utility of AI for pathologists and patients is one of the major current barriers to widespread implementation of AI-assisted pathology tools, highlighting a current area of need in AI and healthcare research [41]. AI has also demonstrated the ability to identify histological findings at levels beyond what the human eye can see, as well as the ability to use genotypic and phenotypic data to more accurately detect the tumour of origin in metastatic cancer [42].

1.6.8 PRIMARY CARE

Primary care has emerged as a critical development area for AI technologies [43, 44]. In primary care, artificial intelligence has been used to aid decision making, predictive modelling, and business analytics [45]. Despite rapid advances in AI technologies, general practitioners' perspectives on the role of AI in primary care are very limited, focusing primarily on administrative and routine documentation tasks [46,47].

1.6.9 PSYCHIATRY

AI applications in psychiatry are still in the proof-of-concept stage [48]. Predictive modelling of diagnosis and treatment outcomes, chatbots, conversational agents that mimic human behaviour and have been studied for anxiety and depression are examples of areas where the evidence is rapidly expanding [49, 50]. One challenge is that many applications in the field are developed and proposed by private corporations, such as Facebook's screening for suicidal ideation in 2017 [51]. Outside of the healthcare system, such applications raise a number of professional, ethical, and regulatory concerns [52]. Another issue that arises frequently is the model's validity and interpretability. Small training datasets contain bias that the models inherit, jeopardising their generalizability and stability. Such models may also be discriminatory toward minority groups that are underrepresented in samples [53].

1.6.10 RADIOLOGY

Artificial intelligence (AI) is being researched in the field of radiology to detect and diagnose diseases using Computerized Tomography (CT) and Magnetic Resonance (MR) Imaging [54]. It may be especially useful in situations where the demand for human expertise exceeds the supply of human experts, or where data is too complex to be efficiently interpreted by human readers [55]. Several deep learning models have demonstrated the ability to be roughly as accurate as healthcare professionals in identifying diseases through medical imaging, though few studies reporting these findings have been externally validated [56]. AI can also benefit radiologists in ways other than interpretation, such as reducing image noise, producing high-quality images with lower doses of radiation, improving MR image quality, and automatically assessing image quality [57]. Further research into the application of AI in nuclear medicine focuses on image reconstruction, anatomical landmarking, and the ability to use lower doses in imaging studies [58].

1.7 CASE STUDIES

The Breast Cancer Wisconsin Diagnostic Data Set was used in this study. The Machine Learning Repository at the University of California, Irvine (UCI) has made this dataset freely available. It is made up of the properties, or features, of cell nuclei extracted from breast tumours using fine-needle aspiration (FNA), a popular oncology diagnostic method. From January 1989 to November 1991, clinical samples were collected for this collection. Relevant features from digitised images of the FNA samples were extracted. An example of one of the digitised images from an FNA sample is given in Figure 1.9 [59].

The primary purpose of illness diagnosis is to determine whether or not a patient is suffering from a disease. Diagnosis may be defined as a "pre-existing set of categories agreed upon by the medical profession to indicate a specific ailment" or as a "process or categorization agreed upon by the medical profession to name a specific illness."

The whole diagnostic process is a sophisticated and "patient-centered, collaborative activity that incorporates information collecting and clinical reasoning with the purpose of diagnosing a patient's health condition," according to the American College of Physicians. To better understand the diagnostic process, the Committee on Diagnostic Error in Health Care established a conceptual model. The patient first has a health problem connected to the individual's symptoms, which leads to the emergence of the illness. individual to contact the healthcare system, where enough information is gathered through a study of the patient's clinical history and an interview, a physical exam and diagnostic tests, and referral and consultation with additional medical professionals. Gathering, integrating, and interpreting data, as well as producing a functioning diagnosis—for example, a single or differential diagnosis-represent a continuous process that may be done several times. The working diagnosis and an explanation of it are shared with the patient, and appropriate treatment is planned. Finally, this process results in an outcome for patients and the healthcare system, such as learning from errors or a timely diagnosis [60]. Figure 1.10 shows the flow of diagnostic process.

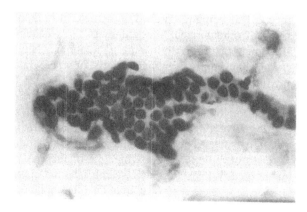

FIGURE 1.9 An image of a breast mass from which dataset features were obtained.

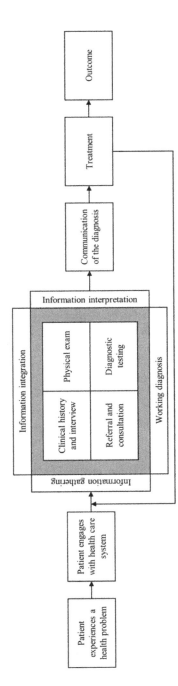

FIGURE 1.10 Flow of diagnostic process.

Machine learning techniques are increasingly being used in healthcare, allowing for more effective estimation and prediction of health outcomes from vast administrative data sets. The study's major goal was to create a general machine learning method for estimating diabetes incidence based on the number of reimbursements during the previous two years. A final data set was picked from a population-based epidemiological cohort (CONSTANCES) connected to the French National Health Database (i.e. SNDS). We used a supervised machine learning method to create this algorithm. The following steps were performed: (i) selection of final data set; (ii) target definition; (iii) Coding variables for a given window of time; (iv) split final data into training and test data sets; (v) variables selection; (vi) training model; (vii) validation of model with test data set; and (viii) Selection of the model. We used the area under the receiver operating characteristic curve (AUC) to select the best algorithm. The final data set used to develop the algorithm included 44,659 participants from CONSTANCES. Out of 3468 variables which were similar to the SNDS and CONSTANCES, cohort were coded and 23 variables used to train multiple algorithms. The final technique for estimating diabetes incidence was a Linear Discriminant Analysis model based on the number of reimbursements for specified variables such as biological testing, medications, medical actions, and hospitalisation without a procedure over the previous two years. This algorithm has a 62% sensitivity, a 67% specificity, and a 67% accuracy. [95% CI: 0.66–0.68] [61].

Dataset is a significant percentage of data since the literature study of AI is gathered during the diagnosis stage of a clinical dataset from electro-diagnosis, diagnosis imaging, and genetic testing. Topol and Jha, for example, encouraged radiologists to use AI technologies to analyse the massive amounts of data retrieved from diagnostic images. There are two additional main data sources: notes taken during physical examinations and results gained from executing lab procedures.

Images, electrophysiological, and genomic datasets can be used to identify physical examination notes and clinical laboratory results since they contain a large number of clinical notes that cannot be analysed directly. As a result, the AI system's primary goal is to turn these unstructured documents into machine-understandable electronic medical data. On the basis of dataset, AI systems are split into two major types. Machine learning techniques are used in the first category to analyse structured data directly. The second group, on the other hand, works on unstructured data utilising natural language processing approaches to improve structured data. For example, in the medical field, machine learning algorithms focus on patient characteristics to cluster them or predict the likelihood of a specific disease, whereas natural language processing aims to convert unstructured data to structured data. Despite growth in the literature on AI in healthcare, the majority of research is focused on a few key illness types such as cancer, cardiovascular disease, and neurological disease. AI in healthcare is still mostly focused on a few diseases, such as cancer, neurological diseases, and cardiovascular disease. These diseases have a significant role in global mortality and require early diagnosis and treatment. Improved analysis procedures are used in this. AI has been used to treat diseases other than the three major ones. Long et al. used ocular imaging data to diagnose congenital cataract illness, and Gulshan et al. used pictures of the retina fundus to detect diabetic retinopathy.

1.8   CURRENT APPLICATIONS OF AI IN MEDICAL DIAGNOSTICS

A sizable portion of today's machine learning analytic applications appears to fit into these categories:

1. Chatbot companies are deploying AI-chatbots with speech recognition features that can discover patterns through symptoms as expressed by the patient in order to draw a possible conclusion, avert disease, and also advise an appropriate course of action.
2. Oncology researchers are attempting to identify malignant tissues using deep learning techniques at a level equivalent to that of a skilled doctor, allowing for detection of cancer in its early stages.
3. Pathology is a vital field that, if covered by AI systems, can be extremely beneficial. It is the science or study of illness origin, nature, and progression as determined by laboratory testing of physiological fluids such as sputum, blood, and urine, as well as tissue analysis. Traditional techniques of diagnosis require the use of a microscope, which can be time-consuming and error-prone. AI technology such as machine learning and machine vision approaches tend to improve pathologists' traditional procedures.

1.9   CONCLUSION

There has been a shift in doctor behaviour from traditional methods to the use of AI chatbots, which are AI versions of doctors. Through the fast-growing fields of machine learning and big data analytics, AI is gaining traction in medical services and is in the process of evolving traditional approaches to diagnosing and treating illnesses. The key to achieving better success in the treatment of disease is early detection. All of this will be impossible to achieve without massive amounts of data, a recognition that AI will complement rather than replace jobs, and a substantial investment in the technology itself. AI is already helping us more efficiently diagnose diseases, develop drugs, personalize treatments, and even edit genes. But this is only the start. The more we digitize and integrate our medical data, the more AI can assist us in identifying useful patterns – patterns that can be used to make correct, cost-effective judgments in complicated analytical procedures.

REFERENCES

1. www.igi-global.com/dictionary/smart-healthcare/76574.
2. S. P. Mohanty, U. Choppali and E. Kougianos, "Everything you wanted to know about smart cities: The Internet of things is the backbone," IEEE Consumer Electronics Magazine, vol. 5, no. 3, pp. 60–70, July 2016.
3. www.tuvsud.com/en/digital-service/smart-healthcare.
4. http://anyk.com/case_view.aspx?TypeId=116&Id=442&FId=t4:116:4.
5. Kashif Hameed, Imran Sarwar Bajwa, Shabana Ramzan, Waheed Anwar and Akmal Khan, An Intelligent IoT Based Healthcare System Using Fuzzy Neural Networks, Scientific Programming, Volume 2020, Article ID 8836927.

6. Prabha Sundaravadivel, Elias Kougianos, Saraju P. Mohanty, and Madhavi K. Ganapathiraju, Everything You wanted to know about smart healthcare, IEEE consumer electronics magazine, January 2018.

7. S. P. Mohanty, Nanoelectronic Mixed-Signal System Design. New York: McGraw-Hill, 2015.

8. A. Bader, H. Ghazzai, A. Kadri, and M. S. Alouini, "Front-end intelligence for large-scale application-oriented internet-of-things," IEEE Access, vol. 4, pp. 3257–3272, June 2016, A. Banerjee and S. K. S. Gupta, "Analysis of smart mobile applications for healthcare under dynamic context changes," IEEE Trans. Mobile Comput., vol. 14, no. 5, pp. 904–919, May 2015.

9. https://searchenterpriseai.techtarget.com/definition/AI-Artificial-Intelligence-Date-19.10.2021.

10. www.visionmonday.com/business/research-and-stats/article/new-benchmark-uspto-study-finds-ai-in-us-patents-rose-by-more-than-100-percent-since-2002-Date19.

11. www.mygreatlearning.com/blog/how-ai-can-improve-healthcare-industry.

12. www.datarevenue.com/en-blog/artificial-intelligence-in-medicine.

13. Wang, Hong; Zu, Quannan; Chen, Jinglu; Yang, Zhiren; Ahmed, Mohammad Anis (October 2021). "Application of Artificial Intelligence in Acute Coronary Syndrome: A Brief Literature Review". Advances in Therapy. 38 (10): 5078–5086.

14. Infante, Teresa; Cavaliere, Carlo; Punzo, Bruna; Grimaldi, Vincenzo; Salvatore, Marco; Napoli, Claudio (December 2021). "Radiogenomics and Artificial Intelligence Approaches Applied to Cardiac Computed Tomography Angiography and Cardiac Magnetic Resonance for Precision Medicine in Coronary Heart Disease: A Systematic Review". Circulation. Cardiovascular Imaging. 14 (12): 1133–1146.

15. Stewart, Jonathon; Lu, Juan; Goudie, Adrian; Bennamoun, Mohammed; Sprivulis, Peter; Sanfillipo, Frank; Dwivedi, Girish (2021). "Applications of machine learning to undifferentiated chest pain in the emergency department: A systematic review". PLOS ONE. 16 (8): e0252612.

16. Sotirakos, Sara; Fouda, Basem; Mohamed Razif, Noor Adeebah; Cribben, Niall; Mulhall, Cormac; O'Byrne, Aisling; Moran, Bridget; Connolly, Ruairi (February 2022). "Harnessing artificial intelligence in cardiac rehabilitation, a systematic review". Future Cardiology. 18 (2): 154–164.

17. Chen, Wei; Sun, Qiang; Chen, Xiaomin; Xie, Gangcai; Wu, Huiqun; Xu, Chen (2021). "Deep Learning Methods for Heart Sounds Classification: A Systematic Review". Entropy. 23 (6): 667.

18. Zhao, Yuan; Wood, Erica P.; Mirin, Nicholas; Cook, Stephanie H.; Chunara, Rumi (October 2021). "Social Determinants in Machine Learning Cardiovascular Disease Prediction Models: A Systematic Review". American Journal of Preventive Medicine. 61 (4): 596–605.

19. Gayathri P, Gopichand G, Geraldine Bessie Amali, Santhi H, A Case Study on Artificial Intelligence Application in Medical Diagnostics, World Wide Journal of Multidisciplinary Research and Development.

20. Hibler, Brian P.; Qi, Qiaochu; Rossi, Anthony M. (March 2016). "Current state of imaging in dermatology". Seminars in Cutaneous Medicine and Surgery. 35 (1): 2–8.

21. Chan, Stephanie; Reddy, Vidhatha; Myers, Bridget; Thibodeaux, Quinn; Brownstone, Nicholas; Liao, Wilson (2020). "Machine Learning in Dermatology: Current Applications, Opportunities, and Limitations". Dermatology and Therapy. 10 (3): 365–386.

22. Han, Seung Seog; Moon, Ik Jun; Lim, Woohyung; Suh, In Suck; Lee, Sam Yong; Na, Jung-Im; Kim, Seong Hwan; Chang, Sung Eun (2020). "Keratinocytic Skin Cancer

Detection on the Face Using Region-Based Convolutional Neural Network". JAMA Dermatology. 156 (1): 29–37.

23. Esteva, Andre; Kuprel, Brett; Novoa, Roberto A.; Ko, Justin; Swetter, Susan M.; Blau, Helen M.; Thrun, Sebastian (February 2017). "Dermatologist-level classification of skin cancer with deep neural networks". Nature. 542 (7639): 115–118.

24. Noyan, Mehmet Alican; Durdu, Murat; Eskiocak, Ali Haydar (2020). "TzanckNet: a convolutional neural network to identify cells in the cytology of erosive-vesiculobullous diseases". Scientific Reports. 10 (1): 18314.

25. Patcas R, Bernini DA, Volokitin A, Agustsson E, Rothe R, Timofte R (January 2019). "Applying artificial intelligence to assess the impact of orthognathic treatment on facial attractiveness and estimated age". International Journal of Oral and Maxillofacial Surgery. 48 (1): 77–83.

26. Patcas R, Timofte R, Volokitin A, Agustsson E, Eliades T, Eichenberger M, Bornstein MM (August 2019). "Facial attractiveness of cleft patients: a direct comparison between artificial-intelligence-based scoring and conventional rater groups". European Journal of Orthodontics. 41 (4): 428–433.

27. "Computer learns to detect skin cancer more accurately than doctors". The Guardian. 29 May 2018.

28. Cao, Jia-Sheng; Lu, Zi-Yi; Chen, Ming-Yu; Zhang, Bin; Juengpanich, Sarun; Hu, Jia-Hao; Li, Shi-Jie; Topatana, Win; Zhou, Xue-Yin; Feng, Xu; Shen, Ji-Liang (2021). "Artificial intelligence in gastroenterology and hepatology: Status and challenges". World Journal of Gastroenterology. 27 (16): 1664–1690.

29. COVID-19 Pandemic Impact: Global R&D Spend for AI in Healthcare and Pharmaceuticals Will Increase US$1.5 Billion By 2025". Medical Letter on the CDC & FDA. May 3, 2020 – via Gale Academic OneFile.

30. Tran, Nam K.; Albahra, Samer; May, Larissa; Waldman, Sarah; Crabtree, Scott; Bainbridge, Scott; Rashidi, Hooman (2021). "Evolving Applications of Artificial Intelligence and Machine Learning in Infectious Diseases Testing". Clinical Chemistry. 68 (1): 125–133.

31. Bhinder, Bhavneet; Gilvary, Coryandar; Madhukar, Neel S.; Elemento, Olivier (April 2021). "Artificial Intelligence in Cancer Research and Precision Medicine". Cancer Discovery. 11 (4): 900–915.

32. Majumder, Anusree; Sen, Debraj (October 2021). "Artificial intelligence in cancer diagnostics and therapy: current perspectives". Indian Journal of Cancer. 58 (4): 481–492.

33. Kobie N (1 January 2020). "DeepMind's new AI can spot breast cancer just as well as your doctor". Wired UK. Wired.

34. McKinney SM, Sieniek M, Godbole V, Godwin J, Antropova N, Ashrafian H, et al. (January 2020). "International evaluation of an AI system for breast cancer screening". Nature. 577 (7788): 89–94.

35. Artificial intelligence identifies prostate cancer with near-perfect accuracy. EurekAlert 27 July 2020.

36. Pantanowitz L, Quiroga-Garza GM, Bien L, Heled R, Laifenfeld D, Linhart C, et al. (1 August 2020). "An artificial intelligence algorithm for prostate cancer diagnosis in whole slide images of core needle biopsies: a blinded clinical validation and deployment study". The Lancet Digital Health. 2 (8): e407–e416.

37. Cao, Jia-Sheng; Lu, Zi-Yi; Chen, Ming-Yu; Zhang, Bin; Juengpanich, Sarun; Hu, Jia-Hao; Li, Shi-Jie; Topatana, Win; Zhou, Xue-Yin; Feng, Xu; Shen, Ji-Liang (2021). "Artificial intelligence in gastroenterology and hepatology: Status and challenges". World Journal of Gastroenterology. 27 (16): 1664–1690.

38. Försch, Sebastian; Klauschen, Frederick; Hufnagl, Peter; Roth, Wilfried (March 2021). "Artificial Intelligence in Pathology". Deutsches Ärzteblatt International. 118 (12): 199–204.

39. Steiner, David F.; MacDonald, Robert; Liu, Yun; Truszkowski, Peter; Hipp, Jason D.; Gammage, Christopher; Thng, Florence; Peng, Lily; Stumpe, Martin C. (December 2018). "Impact of Deep Learning Assistance on the Histopathologic Review of Lymph Nodes for Metastatic Breast Cancer". The American Journal of Surgical Pathology. 42 (12): 1636–1646.

40. Ho, Jonhan; Ahlers, Stefan M.; Stratman, Curtis; Aridor, Orly; Pantanowitz, Liron; Fine, Jeffrey L.; Kuzmishin, John A.; Montalto, Michael C.; Parwani, Anil V. (2014). "Can digital pathology result in cost savings? A financial projection for digital pathology implementation at a large integrated health care organization". Journal of Pathology Informatics. 5 (1): 33.

41. Försch, Sebastian; Klauschen, Frederick; Hufnagl, Peter; Roth, Wilfried (March 2021). "Artificial Intelligence in Pathology". Deutsches Ärzteblatt International. 118 (12): 199–204.

42. Jurmeister, Philipp; Bockmayr, Michael; Seegerer, Philipp; Bockmayr, Teresa; Treue, Denise; Montavon, Grégoire; Vollbrecht, Claudia; Arnold, Alexander; Teichmann, Daniel; Bressem, Keno; Schüller, Ulrich (2019). "Machine learning analysis of DNA methylation profiles distinguishes primary lung squamous cell carcinomas from head and neck metastases". Science Translational Medicine. 11 (509): eaaw8513.

43. Mistry P (September 2019). "Artificial intelligence in primary care". The British Journal of General Practice. 69 (686): 422–423.

44. Blease C, Kaptchuk TJ, Bernstein MH, Mandl KD, Halamka JD, DesRoches CM (March 2019). "Artificial Intelligence and the Future of Primary Care: Exploratory Qualitative Study of UK General Practitioners' Views". Journal of Medical Internet Research. 21 (3): e12802.

45. Liyanage H, Liaw ST, Jonnagaddala J, Schreiber R, Kuziemsky C, Terry AL, de Lusignan S (August 2019). "Artificial Intelligence in Primary Health Care: Perceptions, Issues, and Challenges". Yearbook of Medical Informatics. 28 (1): 41–46.

46. Blease C, Kaptchuk TJ, Bernstein MH, Mandl KD, Halamka JD, DesRoches CM (March 2019). "Artificial Intelligence and the Future of Primary Care: Exploratory Qualitative Study of UK General Practitioners' Views". Journal of Medical Internet Research. 21 (3): e12802.

47. Kocaballi AB, Ijaz K, Laranjo L, Quiroz JC, Rezazadegan D, Tong HL, et al. (November 2020). "Envisioning an artificial intelligence documentation assistant for future primary care consultations: A co-design study with general practitioners". Journal of the American Medical Informatics Association. 27 (11): 1695–1704.

48. Graham S, Depp C, Lee EE, Nebeker C, Tu X, Kim HC, Jeste DV (November 2019). "Artificial Intelligence for Mental Health and Mental Illnesses: An Overview". Current Psychiatry Reports. 21 (11): 116.

49. Chekroud, Adam M.; Bondar, Julia; Delgadillo, Jaime; Doherty, Gavin; Wasil, Akash; Fokkema, Marjolein; Cohen, Zachary; Belgrave, Danielle; DeRubeis, Robert; Iniesta, Raquel; Dwyer, Dominic (2021). "The promise of machine learning in predicting treatment outcomes in psychiatry". World Psychiatry. 20 (2): 154–170.

50. Fulmer R, Joerin A, Gentile B, Lakerink L, Rauws M (December 2018). "Using Psychological Artificial Intelligence (Tess) to Relieve Symptoms of Depression and Anxiety: Randomized Controlled Trial". JMIR Mental Health. 5 (4): e64.

51. Coppersmith G, Leary R, Crutchley P, Fine A (January 2018). "Natural Language Processing of Social Media as Screening for Suicide Risk". Biomedical Informatics Insights. 10: 1178222618792860.

52. Brunn M, Diefenbacher A, Courtet P, Genieys W (August 2020). "The Future is Knocking: How Artificial Intelligence Will Fundamentally Change Psychiatry". Academic Psychiatry. 44 (4): 461–466.

53. Rutledge, Robb B; Chekroud, Adam M; Huys, Quentin JM (2019). "Machine learning and big data in psychiatry: toward clinical applications". Current Opinion in Neurobiology. Machine Learning, Big Data, and Neuroscience. 55: 152–159.

54. Pisarchik AN, Maksimenko VA, Hramov AE (October 2019). "From Novel Technology to Novel Applications: Comment on "An Integrated Brain-Machine Interface Platform with Thousands of Channels" by Elon Musk and Neuralink". Journal of Medical Internet Research. 21 (10): e16356.

55. Hosny A, Parmar C, Quackenbush J, Schwartz LH, Aerts HJ (August 2018). "Artificial intelligence in radiology". Nature Reviews. Cancer. 18 (8): 500–510.

56. Liu, Xiaoxuan; Faes, Livia; Kale, Aditya U; Wagner, Siegfried K; Fu, Dun Jack; Bruynseels, Alice; Mahendiran, Thushika; Moraes, Gabriella; Shamdas, Mohith; Kern, Christoph; Ledsam, Joseph R (2019). "A comparison of deep learning performance against healthcare professionals in detecting diseases from medical imaging: a systematic review and meta-analysis". The Lancet Digital Health. 1 (6): e271–e297.

57. Richardson, Michael L.; Garwood, Elisabeth R.; Lee, Yueh; Li, Matthew D.; Lo, Hao S.; Nagaraju, Arun; Nguyen, Xuan V.; Probyn, Linda; Rajiah, Prabhakar; Sin, Jessica; Wasnik, Ashish P. (September 2021). "Noninterpretive Uses of Artificial Intelligence in Radiology". Academic Radiology. 28 (9): 1225–1235.

58. Seifert, Robert; Weber, Manuel; Kocakavuk, Emre; Rischpler, Christoph; Kersting, David (March 2021). "Artificial Intelligence and Machine Learning in Nuclear Medicine: Future Perspectives". Seminars in Nuclear Medicine. 51 (2): 170–177.

59. Jenni A. M. Sidey-Gibbons1 and Chris J. Sidey-Gibbons, Machine learning in medicine: a practical introduction, BMC Medical Research Methodology (2019) 19:64.

60. Milad Mirbabaie, Stefan Stieglitz, Nicholas R. J. Frick, Artificial intelligence in disease diagnostics: A critical review and classification on the current state of research guiding future direction, Health and Technology (2021) 11:693–731.

61. Romana Haneef, Sofiane Kab, Rok Hrzic, Sonsoles Fuentes, Sandrine Fosse-Edorh, Emmanuel Cosson and Anne Gallay, Use of artificial intelligence for public health surveillance: a case study to develop a machine Learning-algorithm to estimate the incidence of diabetes mellitus in France, Haneef et al. Archives of Public Health (2021) 79:168.

2 Securing IoT Devices for Healthcare Systems Using Optimization-Based Approaches

Ankur Khare,[1] Rajendra Gupta,[1] and Piyush Shukla[2]
[1] Rabindra Nath Tagore University, Raisen, Bhopal, Madhya Pradesh, India
[2] Rajiv Gandhi Technical University, Bhopal, Madhya Pradesh, India

CONTENTS

2.1 INTRODUCTION

WSN (Wireless sensor network) is an amalgamation of numerous tiny nodes known as IoT devices, having sensors that are emerging in a 5G environment area that is easily affected by malicious users. Sensors are basically small devices with the ability to sense, record and process the information. Sensor networks are present everywhere [58]. They are meant for measuring physical parameters like pressure, sound, temperature, chemical composition, etc. Each sensor contains components

DOI: 10.1201/9781003145035-2

like transceiver, microcontroller, external memory, power source, etc. Due to ease of deployment and inexpensive nature of sensor nodes, WSN is utilized in many important applications like armed forces and security applications, seismic monitoring, health monitoring, industrialized automation, robust monitoring, etc. The healthcare WSN is considered as a broad area of research because many critical applications in healthcare settings directly or indirectly depend upon sensor networks [22]. IoT devices communicate through various routing protocols. Nodes with sensing capacity may be itinerant and motionless. Itinerant sensor nodes can communicate through MANETs (Mobile Ad-hoc Networks). IoT devices are disseminated in an area communicating through multiple hops with each other by forwarding data packets in MANETs [39].

Due to the increase in the dependability of sensor networks, there is a decrease in the security of medical data. Sensor networks are easily affected by attackers as they have fewer security mechanisms [27]. Security is a major concern as any malicious user can misuse critical information by launching dangerous types of attacks like passive attack [18], routing attack [18], active attack [18], denial of service attack [3], node replication attack, spoofing attack, etc. Thus, there is a need to equip sensor networks with security mechanisms instruct to ensure discretion, veracity, and authenticity of medical information in IoT environments [33].

Main features of this technology includes: a few or large number of nodes having asymmetric data surge commencing nodes to a instruct node having sensing capability and communication is initiated by actions in 5G. Every node performs broadcast message passing if there is sufficient power capability [27]. All IoT devices have sensing capability but not all are globally identified for worldwide communication. The network architecture depends on the application deploying the IoT WSN. For example, some IoT devices are linked directly to the sink without passing via former nodes. Other layers might go through other nodes to forward the data to the sink [12].

The small-sized nodes have inherent limitations and thus privacy is a crucial concern in IoT WSNs. Such networks are insecure due to malicious and substantial attacks by means of transmission, untrusted communication, and neglected scenery [12]. The sensors in IoT devices have inadequate strength; therefore it is very exigent to offer security to IoT devices with storage, energy, and computation requirement. Consequently, several enhancements in IoT WSN like epidemic methodology [52], UML (unified modelling language) methods [56, 57], vulnerability evaluations, and probabilistic analysis have been developed to overcome the limitations of sensor IoT devices to resist against the node capture attack. In certain modelling methods, the attacker randomly captures node to compromise in the communication of a whole sensor network. However, vulnerability evaluation approach has been formalized whereby an attacker can select a node intelligently to compromise the network using vulnerability metric [11]. The main objective of this chapter is to discuss different types of attacks and security issues and the optimization approaches used to resist node capture attacks on IoT devices in healthcare environments. Another objective is to describe how to enhance the optimization approaches based on security, toughness and running time for military and medical applications. This chapter also explains how to increase the privacy of IoT devices [16].

2.2 IOT-BASED WIRELESS SENSOR NETWORKS

Wireless sensor networks (WSNs) are one of the most fundamental technologies of the Internet of Things (IoT) for sensing, communicating and reputing among nodes. Therefore, numerous fields utilize WSN for medication, transportation, agriculture, process management and ecological discipline [26]. In fact, the world looks forward to simplifying complex problems than just operating the thermostat through mobile. Smart homes, smart buildings, smart cities, smart agriculture, and supply chain management are just a few of the areas that the wireless sensor networks will dramatically impact. The distinguishing traits of WSN have a straight brunt on structural node`s model with few levels: command resource, processor, communication structure, and sensors [35, 57].

2.2.1 STRUCTURE OF IoT-WSNs

WSNs are an emerging area that consists of multiple IoT devices (either mobile or static), a sink station, wireless medium, and a base station (task manager) in IoT environments [12, 16]. The components of IoT-WSN are described in the following and shown in Figure 2.1:

- **Sensor field**: A sensor field is like a coverage area such as a forest, ocean, home, etc., in which sensors are deployed in a distributed manner [16].
- **Sensor node**: This is a miniature machine or IoT device that contains four components: transceiver, power source, microcontroller, sensing unit, and processor. IoT devices collect, process, and record all the data traffic that is communicated through the whole network [21, 23].
- **Sink**: The sink is the point where every IoT device forwards the collected healthcare data, which is later aggregated in order to start communication with the sink station [12].

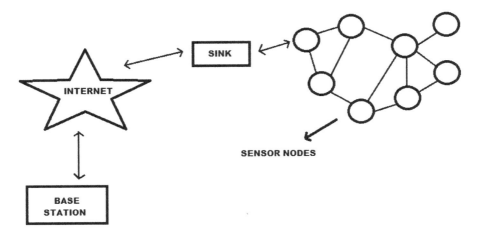

FIGURE 2.1 Structure of IoT-WSNs.

- **Base station**: This is the edge point between the end users and the network. It provides all the services to the user according to their requirements. It manages all the communication tasks between the sensor nodes or IoT devices. Thus, it is also called the task manager [14].

2.2.2 CHARACTERISTICS OF IoT-WSNs

The important characteristics of IoT-WSNs are as follows:

- **Scalability**: Sensor networks possess dynamic topology in which we can either increase or decrease the number of sensor nodes (IoT devices). Thus, 5G-WSNs are scalable enough to handle a large number of sensors [2].
- **Resilience**: IoT-WSNs are highly resilient and provide an immediate service if any fault or node failure occurs within the network. They have the ability to cope with all the structural changes that do not affect the normal operation of IoT devices [18].
- **Self-organized**: The randomly deployed IoT devices can adjust easily and work in a cooperative manner. IoT devices may be mobile or static depending upon whether we are using an ad-hoc network or not. They tend to communicate with each other by forwarding the data packets of healthcare systems in an organized way from one hop to another [9, 18].
- **Multi-hop communication**: Sensor nodes (IoT devices) transmit the data packets of healthcare systems through the multiple hops present among sources and destinations. In this way, every IoT device checks the authenticity of the medical data packet and then forwards it to the subsequent hop until the data packet reaches to its destination node securely [39].
- **Application-oriented**: Due to its very nature, IoT-WSNs can be effectively used for application-oriented problems. The deployment of the IoT devices done accordingly and its behaviour vary from application to application [54, 55].

2.2.3 CHALLENGES OF IoT-WSNs

The major challenges of IoT-WSNs are as follows:

- **Real-time operation**: Most critical applications of IoT-WSNs deal with real-time environments. Successful transmission of medical data packets in real time is somewhat difficult. Message loss by intermediate nodes, congestion, disturbing noise, and other transmission problems delay the operation of IoT devices. Thus, the delivery of packets cannot be done in time, which is the main challenge in WSNs [18].
- **Security**: Maintaining the security in WSNs is the biggest challenge. IoT networks are developed in an environment where they can easily be affected by malicious activities. There should be security methods associated with every sensor node [19].

- **Unreliable communication**: All the medical data packets are broadcasted through multiple hops with connectionless routing protocols for large distances. In this way communication between nodes is not reliable. Thus, there is a need to use connection-oriented protocols [9].
- **Energy**: Maintaining the overall energy of a sensor network is a big challenge. Every sensor node has its own energy, which is consumed when the node transmits the medical data packets. If there are large numbers of sensors, then more energy is required [18]. There may be the case when regular power becomes low or negligible. Thus, there should be technology that works in the area of energy utilization of IoT-WSNs [1].

2.2.4 SECURITY CONCERNS IN IoT-WSNs

WSNs are prone to attacks and the broadcast nature of broadcast standards makes them vulnerable to attacks [18]. While talking about security, we need to talk about the following security concerns (Figure 2.2):

- **Data authentication**: This is the procedure of identification and verification of a system's users and the IoT device that checks the authenticity of users [54]. It is provided a document validation and verification utilizing the digital credentials. It can be used to identify in the IoT WSN whether healthcare information is coming from an authenticated user or not [29, 38].
- **Data flexibility**: Data is flexible for all users in a network providing full access and control on medical data information flowing among IoT devices

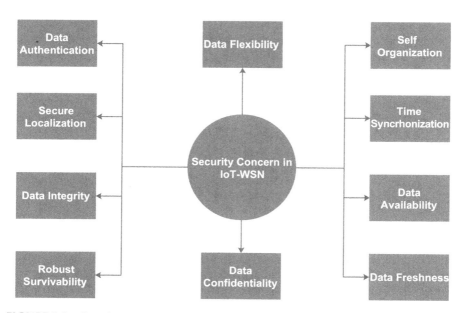

FIGURE 2.2   Security concerns in 5G-WSN.

in IoT-WSNs [54]. Data flexibility provides facilities to users to interchange, submit and retrieve their documents easily in IoT-WSN.

- **Self-organization**: IoT devices are structured and controlled by their own set of rules and regulations. Self-organized IoT devices communicate with each other in IoT-WSNs and perform functions like synchronization, routing, power consumption, and secure message passing [1, 18].
- **Secure localization**: Attackers aim to capture unknown IoT devices that are located in IoT-WSNs. Secure localization is provided to unknown IoT devices to protect them from attackers. Localization is becoming very important in secure medical and military applications to ensure authenticated positions of all IoT devices [18].
- **Time synchronization**: IoT devices are synchronized with each other to allow communication in a secure IoT-WSN. This is also necessary for well utilization of all active and passive IoT devices and for monitoring, hustle assessment, intention tracking, and incident exposure [18].
- **Data integrity**: It is surety of exact information transmission, which is not modified or altered by attacker when medical information is passing through medium. It is obtained using authentication because wrong healthcare data creates confusion and generates the harmful effects on data transmission with false decisions [1, 38].
- **Data availability**: Data availability in IoT devices is intended to provide accessibility of data at all times without regarding network disruptions due to influence levels, machine drops, and machine modification, etc. It also provides resistance against several attacks. Public data availability is more important to resist against node capture attacks [1, 18].
- **Robust survivability**: WSNs is survivable against attacks such as node capture threat, key compromise, etc. If single or multiple IoT devices are controlled by an attacker then whole IoT-WSN is survivable or not destroyed. Machine survivability is the strength to complete its tasks, in sensible approach in the occurrence of failures, active and passive attacks [18].
- **Data confidentiality**: Healthcare information is confidentially transmitted to the receiver, and the message is received by the actual receiver not other nodes. It is achieved by encrypting the information using a public key of receivers so encrypted message is decrypted by using receiver's private key. This maintains the secrecy of medical information [1, 18].
- **Data freshness**: Data freshness is directly related to the latest medical information, which is updated and modified in real time. The fresh data is provided to the IoT devices for time synchronization (strong freshness) and sensing procedure (weak freshness) in IoT-WSNs [1, 38].

2.3 TYPES OF ATTACKS ON IOT-WSNS

Healthcare information is transferred over IoT-WSNs using broadcasting, which provides an easy way to seize or interrupt information transmission among IoT devices [3]. The attacker generates the interruptions in the services of IoT-WSN. Attacks are classified and discussed in the following and shown in basis (Figure 2.3).

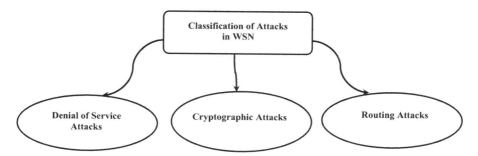

FIGURE 2.3   Classification of attacks.

2.3.1   DENIAL OF SERVICE (DOS) ATTACKS

IoT devices or the whole IoT-WSN is shut down or crashed due to heavy traffic sent by the attacker in a DoS attack. The banking sector, government organizations, finance companies, and share markets are mainly targeted in this type of attack [3]. Secret medical information and cost-related data are the main targets. Flooding and crashing are two basic types of DoS attack. A lot of traffic coming from clients' IoT devices to the server is targeted in a flooding attack, so the speed of the server is slow and the server can crash. This results in the loss of private and important healthcare information from the server. In crashing, the attacker uses the vulnerabilities of IoT devices, including bugs and weak points. Another type of DoS attack is called a SYN flood in which the attacker rapidly initiates a connection without finalizing the connection [3].

A DDoS (Distributed Denial of Service) attack is a specific category of DoS attack in which several IoT devices devise a harmonized DoS attack on a particular object [32]. In this type of attack the attacker attacks from various positions rather than a single position. The attacker can utilize numerous IoT devices to accomplish the attack. The attacker position is also complicated to discover because of arbitrarily allocated IoT devices in IoT-WSNs [32].

2.3.2   CRYPTOGRAPHIC ATTACKS

Cryptographic attacks are usually characterized as active and passive depending upon the attacker exploitation [18].

- **Passive attacks** are usually initiated to steal information by unauthorized access to IoT devices. They do not modify or alter the information and communication medium. They are more dangerous than other attacks because the user does not get informed about the attack [1].
- **Active attacks** are usually used to update or alter data by unauthorized access to IoT devices. The attacker controls the user IoT device and modifies or deletes important information from it [18].

There is further characterization of cryptographic attacks on the basis of attacking manner, methodology, or structure. The main aim of a cryptographic attack is to discover encryption keys and plaintext from cipher text as well [59].

- **Cipher text only attack** – an attack in which attackers have several cipher texts to find out the keys and plain text [59].
- **Known plaintext attack** – an attack in which attackers have only a few plain texts to evaluate the encryption keys and remaining plain text from cipher text [59].
- **Chosen plaintext attack** – an attack in which attackers choose arbitrary plaintext and its corresponding ciphertext to acquire the secret encryption key for next cipher text for future transmission [59].
- **Brute force attack** – an attack in which the attackers apply all possible combinations of keys. It means the total possible combinations of keys are 65536 for 16-bit long keys ($2^{16}=65536$) [3].
- **Timing attack** – an attack in which the attacker identifies the manner of computation. Thus if the encryption key size is larger, the encryption process is longer [7, 43].
- **Power analysis attack** – an attack that uses power expenditure for utilizing encryption to generate useful information for attackers [18].

2.3.3 ROUTING ATTACKS

Routing attacks are network layer attacks in which the router is injected with malicious codes when information is transferred among IoT devices in WSN [18]. Some of the most common router attacks generally include:

- **Black-hole attack**: In this type of attack, a malicious device (black hole) attack the entire traffic having smallest route in IoT-WSN. When a black hole receives a request packet from its neighbour's then malicious message is sent by black hole to know about the route of packets transmission [30]. Thus, neighboring IoT devices are modified their routing tables with black hole details.
- **Wormhole attack**: In this type of attack, the attacker captures the packets or bits of packets at one place and forwards the packet to another malicious node at the other end of the network through a tunnel. As a result the other nodes in the network can be tricked into believing that they are near to other nodes which can cause problems in the routing algorithm [49].
- **Grey-hole attack**: In this type of attack, a malicious node may constantly or randomly drop packets and therefore reduce the efficiency of the networking system. [48].
- **Node capture attack**: In this type of attack, an intruder captures the IoT devices and controls the entire IoT-WSN [24]. The intruder takes out the necessary information such as encryption keys and routing procedures from the IoT devices in the IoT-WSNs. Two IoT devices are communicated with each other if they used some common keys in their transmission ranges [10, 11]. It is difficult to determine which IoT devices are controlled by the

attacker due to the large of IoT-WSNs. The various properties of IoT devices such as mobility, location, energy, and contribution are utilized to obtain the optimal nodes controlling in IoT-WSN [18]. On the basis of these properties the attacker determines the nodes to be attacked to compromise the IoT-WSN.

2.4 OPTIMIZATION TECHNIQUES AND FUNCTIONS

Optimization is a process of obtaining the optimal solution from the set of the possible solutions on the basis of some specific condition. Objective functions are functions that minimize or maximize the overall function value based on some constraints in place of some solution [8, 28]. Further optimization generates the most appropriate function value surrounded by a specified area. Optimization is a tactic, proceed or procedure or of creating incredible as copious ideal, useful, or effectual as feasible [17].

The simplification of optimization assumption and approaches to further examinations comprises a huge region of functional arithmetic. Further, optimization adds obtaining best possible standards of objective function agreed a distinct province (constraints group), examining a multiplicity of unusual characteristics of objective functions and diverse categories of region [8, 34].

The optimization problem has the following major elements:

- **Objective function**: one or more elements (variables) are combined to form a single or multi-objective function to generate a minimum or maximum value with few constraints [53]. Different elements are not attuned with each other or given distinct results, so some weight factors are combined with these elements to form objective functions to provide optimal results [6, 8].
- **Variables**: one or more unknown elements necessary for the objective function are denoted as variables. Variables are utilized to explain a single or multi-objective function and attain some specific conditions and serviceable requirements. They are continuous or discrete based on the problems and constraints [7, 17].
- **Constraints**: they are the set of specific rules that provide particular values to the variables which prevents us from going forever in certain directions. Generally there are some situations in which the objective function is generated with the help of variables. Objective function, variables, and constraints are merged to describe the optimization problem [8, 42].

2.5 EXPLANATION OF APPROACHES AND OPTIMIZATION METHODS FOR NODE CAPTURE ATTACKS

The security of WSNs can be compromised by attackers which gain control of IoT devices and communication mediums and generate interruptions in packet delivery like updating or deleting the packets. A sensor device broadcasts HELLO packets to all other devices for establishing communication. Thus, there is a greater chance to attack these flooding packets among devices. This type of attack is known as the HELLO flood attack. It is defended against using bidirectional verification between two neighboring nodes sharing some protocol. The protocol provides secure communication between two IoT devices excluding all other devices in the WSN. This process can be adopted for IoT devices in WSNs to provide resistance against the HELLO flood attack [31]. Another threat to WSNs is known as the Denial of Service (DoS) attack, which is initiated against IoT devices to capture and destroy the network. The attacker sends several connection requests to the server to slow it down and eventually stop it. A deep learning methodology using a neural network has been designed and applied to detect DoS attack and reduce its effects [37]. The DoS attack is easily launched in distributed WSN which is complicated to identify and tough to protect. It is a Distributed DoS (DDoS) attack in which a clone node or attacker node sends various requests through the clients to the server. The server receives these requests and keeps busy on replying the clients and leaves the main process. The speed of the server is slowly reduced and the server may crash after some time. A Fuzzy Guard is a fuzzy inference system to detect and prevent against DDoS attack by utilizing autonomous routing mechanism. Several possible inhibition levels are applied consequently to compact with flood of attack to economically decrease the attack collision on WSN in IoT environment. The Fuzzy Guard approach could be prevented the packet flooding in attacking level and defended against DDoS attack with less communication overhead and resource expenditure [32].

A sensor IoT node is good or bad; it is decided by its trust value which is evaluated on the basis of historical medical information about misbehavior of that sensor node in IoT-WSN. The attacker nodes are detected using an O2Trust method to provide the trust value for every node, so the good nodes are selected for communication rather than the bad nodes. This helps for future selection of sensor nodes based on trust value with On-Off attack improvement [36]. The misbehavior of sensor nodes is also shown by selective forwarding attack, which can be accurately detected using an E-watchdog method with minimum energy expenditure. The strength of attack detection is enhanced effectively due to selection of detector nearest the attacker. False information coming from attacker node is exempted by an election process to decrease the forged detection rate and enhance the strength of detection with minimum power expenditure [47].

Another selective forwarding attack is grey-hole attack, which is a specific kind of DoS attack. The grey-hole attack affects secrecy, integrity, and accessibility of data in WMNs and damages the whole network by destroying sensitive information. A specific technique called FADE (Forwarding Assessment-based Detection) was developed to fight grey-hole attack. Furthermore, FADE preserves coexistence with existing connection protection approaches. The optimal recognition threshold is examined to reduce the forged positive and negative rate of FADE with corrupted medium quality in WMNs [48]. The attacker changes the traffic from one portion to another in WSNs by adding a minimum cost channel between two portions. This kind of attack is known as a wormhole attack. A DIDS (Distributed Intrusion Detection System) is introduced to watch and detect wormhole attacks in WSNs. The attacked channel is detected using an intrusion system based on criteria like minimum energy and cost [49].

Various real-time applications like Unmanned Aerial Vehicles (UAVs), IoT devices, and automatic cars use an ROS (Robot Operating System). Robotic camera photos can be flown without security. This privacy is generated by using some assessment on security and the uneven flow of unsecure information is detected by intrusion detection system. Image comparisons are performed and abnormal data flows can be detected by ROS. The image comparison experiments are performed on robotic cameras in automatic cars [55]. The intruder introduces an attack to obtain replicas of IoT sensor nodes in IoT-WSN; this is known as a node replication attack. It is very complex and tough to find these replicas in networks due to high mobility of sensor nodes. In view of the restrictions of centralized recognition methods for stationary WSN, some dispersed methodologies have been developed to find replication attacks. Movable nodes ID and various positions are used for hybrid local and comprehensive recognition approaches. Local recognition is applied in local fields and global recognition is initiated in global fields to enhance selection of malicious nodes with replicas [60].

Another hybrid approach based on Danger Theory (DT) is combining the centralized and distributed approach to detect and prevent replication attack in WSNs. The several steps performed to detect replication attack in DT are.; firstly the nature of nodes examine, after that power examine and at last information provide to WSN [51]. The efficiency of this hybrid approach is analyzed in terms of power, time, and delay of detection, overhead, and false negatives. This approach combines all the features and overcomes the disadvantages of centralized and distributed detection methods [20]. The purposes of WSN illustration study is to determine the small dimensional sensor node generation that confine grid organization and are helpful for resolving various problems. Still, regardless of the explosion of these approaches there is presently nothing to describe robustness to adversarial attacks. The vulnerability examination is broadly used arbitrary walks for attacker perturbations [4].

WSNs are susceptible to node capture attacks due to development of IoT devices in communication environment unattended,. Formerly intruder seizes nodes and compromises the WSN by attacking through node capture attacks. Consequently, node capture attacks are perilous and ought to be detected in minimum time to decrease the damage done by attacker. A sequential analysis is applied to detect this type of attack [25]. The identification of node capture attack is extremely difficult in heterogeneous wireless ad hoc networks. Some of the traditional adversarial approaches have been found to be inappropriate for attacks due to overhead cost of capturing and mobility of sensor IoT devices. The low cost and high probabilistic detection of node capture attack is performed by using integer programming concepts based on attacker`s knowledge descriptions and some greedy heuristics approaches applied for minimum power expenditure to identify the limit of network compromise. Individual sensor node memory modification is used to diminish the consequences of attacks using security keeping protocols [39].

The attacker model for finding the node capture attack in WSN yielding the minimum cost can be formulated as an integer-programming minimization problem. Various constraint matrices are introduced in some decomposition methods for node capture attack protection models [41]. In meticulous, an imperative difficulty in the extremely dispersed and reserve inhibited situation is node capture by intruder for modification and stealing the information of sensor nodes. Although widespread effort has been made toward manipulative approaches for protecting and hindrance node compromise or sensible recognize and rescind captured sensor nodes. Stimulated by newly arrived attacks scattering over atmosphere interfaces, epidemic theory is utilized to detect node compromise in WSNs. The pairwise key approach and topological distinctiveness is well formed for defense strategies against large-scale node capture attack [44].

The node capture attack is not completely removed from the WSN, but it is minimized to reduce the impact. The maximum node density and neighborhood contribution are influencing factors to form vulnerabilities in WSN. These vulnerabilities are used by intruders for attacking the network and misusing the secret information of IoT devices. A probabilistic model with hash chain approach is applied on the network to reduce the chance of attack and also to detect the compromised nodes at a higher level. Each node has a hash chain to evaluate the misbehavior of that node, which provides information on whether the node is compromised or not [45]. Some researchers have also developed a few approaches to enhance the efficiency and performance of node capture attack with minimum resource consumption. It has been achieved by developing a GNRMK (Greedy Node capture based on Route Minimum Key set) approach, which evaluates the number of keys in every route to generate a key-route association with higher flow in a WSN. The node is captured on the basis of key-route association value with higher overlapping. GNRMK determines the lowest number of nodes to compromise entire WSN [19].

Table 2.1 gives a comparative analysis of various research works.

RA (Random Attack) is used to select the sensor nodes randomly in every repetition [13, 15]. The number of keys is used for detecting nodes to be captured; it is known as MKA (Maximum Key Attack) [13, 46]. The number of links among sensor nodes is used to discover the probable captured sensor nodes; it is called MLA (Maximum Link Attack) [14, 15]. Similarly the compromised traffic ratio is used to obtain the possible compromised sensor nodes, which is known as MTA (Maximum Traffic Attack) [13, 15]. GNAVE (Greedy Node capture Approximation using Vulnerability Evaluation) is another way to use vulnerabilities of IoT-WSNs to identify probable captured nodes [14, 40]. Another approach implemented to enhance the efficiency of node capture attack is Matrix Algorithm (MA), which is an attacker model with minimum resource consumption and higher reliability. The relationship among keys and paths in WSNs are evaluated and then path-key association is obtained. At last both are combined to form node-path association. The cost of every sensor node is evaluated on the basis of direct and indirect association among nodes and paths. Finally the nodes can be captured based on the node cost. MA shows the minimum nodes captured with the maximum compromised traffic and minimum resource consumption in the most effective time over WSN as compared to the RA, MKA, MKA, MTA and GNAVE [14].

An enhanced form of MA has been developed with minimum resource consumption, which is known as MREA (Minimum Resource Expenditure node capture Attack). A NP-Hard problem is obtained by converting the set covering to the Hamiltonian cycle problem to find the shortest path for reducing the transferring cost in IoT-WSNs. MREA has generate improved results due to evaluation of the shortest path with less resource consumption [13]. Attacking efficiency with minimum execution time is further enhanced by introducing another approach called FGA (Full

TABLE 2.1
Comparative Analysis of Various Works of Researchers

Authors	Node Selection Method	Network Type	Type of Attack	Advantages	Remark
A. Bojchevski et.al. [4]	Eigenvalue perturbation theory	Mobile Centralized	Poisoning Attack	Minimum Memory Complexity	Maximum Communication expenditure
A. Khare et.al. [5]	GWOA multi-objective function	Mobile Centralized	Node Capture Attack	Minimum Communication Overhead	Enhanced Detection rate
A. Khare et.al. [6]	DOA multi-objective function	Mobile Centralized	Node Capture Attack	Balanced Throughput	Single Point Failure
C. Lin et.al. [13]	MREA	Static Centralized	Node Capture Attack	Minimum Overhead	Appropriate for mobile WSN
C. Lin et.al. [14]	MA	Static Distributed	Node Capture Attack	Minimum Memory Complexity	Enhanced Detection rate
C. Lin et.al. [15]	PCA and OGA	Mobile Centralized	Node Capture Attack	Balanced Throughput	Maximum Detection rate
G. Wu et.al. [19]	GNRMK	Mobile Distributed	Node Capture Attack	Average Memory Overhead	Minimum Resource Expenditure
H. R. Shaukat et.al. [20]	Multi-level replica detection using danger theory	Static Distributed	Clone Attack	Minimum Memory Complexity	Maximum Detection rate
J. W. Ho [25]	SPRT	Mobile Distributed	Node Capture Attack	Minimum Delay, Highly Secure	Average Detection Possibility
M. A. Hamid et.al. [31]	Probabilistic secret sharing protocol with bidirectional verification	Mobile Centralized	HELLO Flood Attack	Minimum Communication Overhead	Reduce Vulnerability
M. Huang et.al. [32]	Fuzzy Guard	Mobile Distributed	DDoS attack	Minimum Overhead	Minimum Resource Expenditure
N. Labraoui et.al. [36]	O²Trust	Mobile Distributed	On-Off Attack	Maximum Detection Possibility	Enhanced detection rate

(continued)

TABLE 2.1 (Continued)
Comparative Analysis of Various Works of Researchers

Authors	Node Selection Method	Network Type	Type of Attack	Advantages	Remark
O. Brun et.al. [37]	Deep Learning	Statically Centralized	DoS Attack	Average Memory Overhead	Single Point Failure
P. Tague et.al. [39]	Greedy Heuristic Approach	Mobile Centralized	Node Capture Attack	Minimum Overhead	Single Point Failure
P. Tague et.al. [41]	Heuristic Algorithm	Static Centralized	Node Capture Attack	Maximum Security	Enhanced detection rate
P. K. Shukla et.al. [42]	PSO and GA multi-objective function	Mobile Distributed	Node Capture Attack	Maximum Security	Average Detection Possibility
P. De et.al. [44]	Epidemic Theory	Mobile Distributed	Node Capture Attack	Minimum Communication Overhead	Reduce Vulnerability
P. Ahlawat et.al. [45]	Hash Chain Method	Static Centralized	Node Capture Attack	Minimum Delay, Highly Secure	Average Detection Possibility
Q. Zhang et.al. [47]	E-watchdog	Mobile Distributed	Forwarding Attack	Maximum Security	Enhanced Detection rate
Q. Liu et.al. [48]	FADE	Mobile Distributed	Grey Hole Attack	Average Memory Overhead	Maximum Detection rate
R. D. Graaf et.al. [49]	Distributed Intrusion detection System	Mobile Centralized	Wormhole Attack	Minimum Communication Overhead	Reduce Vulnerability
R. Bhatt et.al. [50]	FFOA multi-objective function	Static Centralized	Node Capture Attack	Average Memory Overhead	Appropriate for mobile WSN
S. Lagraa et.al. [55]	ROS	Mobile Distributed	Real-time Attack	Minimum Memory Complexity	Maximum Detection rate
Z. wang et.al. [60]	Hybrid Detection Method	Mobile Distributed	Node Replication Attack	Minimum Communication Overhead	Reduce Vulnerability

Graph Attack), which captures the sensor nodes on the basis of destructiveness degree of nodes. Additionally the efficiency of FGA is increased by using optimization approaches such as OGA (Opti-Graph Attack) and PCA (Path Covering Attack). The graph of a FGA is optimized using OGA and the shortest path is evaluated using PCA. The energy expenditure and attacking times are reduced and attacking efficiency is increased for OGA, PCA and FGA as compared to other approaches [15].

The only energy is not suitable for selection of nodes to be captured; other factors like node contribution and key utilization are also utilized to compromise the sensor IoT nodes in WSNs. Multiple objectives such as energy cost, participation of sensor nodes, and key utilization are combined to evaluate the nodes' importance values. After that an optimization approach such as FiRAO-PG (Finding Robust Assailant Optimization Particle swarm optimization and Genetic algorithm) is applied on this multi-objective function to obtain optimal value for selection of compromised sensor nodes. The features of PSO (Particle Swarm Optimization) and GA (Genetic Algorithm) are combined to generate the optimal value of the multi-objective function, which is further utilized for selection of probable captured sensor nodes. FiRAO-PG shows higher attacking efficiency than MA in terms of compromised traffic fraction [42]. FFOA (Fruit Fly Optimization Algorithm) is another popular optimization technique that is applied using the multi-objective function that combines the sensor node and key participation and resource expenditure to identify optimal sensor nodes in WSNs. It will manipulate a comprehensive device to knock down utmost division of the WSN beside by way of effectual cost and greatest offensive competence. The FFOA generates improved efficiency in terms of fraction compromised traffic, attacking time, and cost of energy over WSNs compared to GA and other approaches [50].

A GWOA (Grey Wolf Optimization Algorithm) was developed to determine the sensor nodes with the greatest opportunity of being attacked in WSN. GWOA implements an multi-objective function combining several factors such as stability and participation of sensor nodes. The stability is evaluated on the basis of velocity and location of sensor nodes. Sensor node participation is evaluated on the basis of neighborhood degree (number of neighbors of sensor nodes). GWOA shows superior competence in terms of attacking rounds, power cost, and traffic compromised against ACO (Ant Colony Optimization) and other approaches [5]. A DOA (Dragonfly Optimization Algorithm) is implemented to identify the sensor nodes that have the best chance of being attacked in WSN. DOA uses a multi-objective function that merges various factors such as power cost, key utilization, and node velocity. Power cost is calculated using direct and indirect association of sensor nodes. Key utilization calculates the number of keys for each sensor node. Velocity is directly associated with mobility of sensor nodes. DOA shows the superior competence based on attacking rounds, energy cost, and compromised fraction against PSO and other techniques [6].

Table 2.2 gives a comparative analysis of several node capture approaches.

2.6   CONCLUSIONS AND FUTURE DIRECTIONS

IoT-WSNs are self-organizing, self-repairing, and operate a dynamic topology in the multi-hop environment, which faults tolerance and vulnerability to malicious attacks. IoT devices have stored the information by using sensors on them. The

TABLE 2.2
Comparative Analysis of Several Node Capture Approaches

Approach	Node Selection Method	Network Type	Memory Cost	Advantages	Remark
RA [13]	Randomly	Statically Centralized	$O(1)$	Minimum Communication Overhead	Reduce Vulnerability
MKA [14]	Key-based selection	Static Centralized	$O(N^2)$	Minimum Communication Overhead	Maximum Detection rate
MLA [15]	Links-based selection	Static Centralized	$O(N^4)$	Minimum Memory Complexity	Appropriate for mobile WSN
MTA [13]	Traffic-based selection	Static Distributed	$O(N^2)$	Minimum Memory Complexity	Appropriate for mobile WSN
GNAVE [14]	Greedy Vulnerability Evaluation	Mobile Centralized	$O(N^5)$	Average Memory Overhead	Maximum Detection rate
MA [14]	Key Sharing between nodes and paths	Mobile Distributed	$O(N^2)$	Average Memory Overhead	Single Point Failure
PCA [15]	Parameter Destructive rank	Static Distributed	$O(N^2)$	Minimum Overhead	Maximum Detection rate
FGA [15]	Graph and Traffic-based selection	Mobile Centralized	$O(N^2)$	Minimum Overhead	Maximum Detection rate
OGA [15]	Optimized Graph-based selection	Mobile Centralized	$O(N^2)$	Minimum Memory Complexity	Enhanced detection rate
MREA [13]	Heuristic Algorithm	Mobile Distributed	$O(N^2)$	Average Memory Overhead	Minimum Resource Expenditure
ACO [5]	ACO applied on multi-objective function (Stability and node contribution)	Mobile Distributed	$O(N^2)$	Minimum Delay, Highly Secure	Average Detection Possibility

PSO [6]	PSO applied on multi-objective function (velocity, Key and energy expenditure)	Mobile Distributed	$O(N^2)$	Minimum Delay, Highly Secure	Average Detection Possibility
GWOA [5]	GWOA applied on multi-objective function (Stability and node contribution)	Mobile Distributed	$O(N^2)$	Maximum Security	Enhanced Detection rate
DOA [6]	PSO applied on multi-objective function (velocity, Key and energy expenditure)	Mobile Distributed	$O(N^2)$	Maximum Security	Enhanced Detection rate
GA [50]	GA applied on multi-objective function (cost, Key and vertex participation)	Mobile Distributed	$O(N^3)$	Balanced Throughput	Enhanced Detection rate
FiRAO-PG [42]	PSO and GA applied on multi-objective function (cost, Key and route-node participation)	Mobile Distributed	$O(N^3)$	Maximum Detection Possibility	Maximum Communication expenditure
FFOA [50]	FFOA applied on multi-objective function (cost, Key and vertex participation)	Mobile Distributed	$O(N^2)$	Maximum Security	Enhanced Detection rate

sensor IoT device can sense on the basis of temperature and pressure. These devices are utilized for various real-life applications in medical and military environments. Due to numerous applications of IoT devices, it is important and necessary to protect these devices from capture by attackers, which use the IoT devices to steal private information or to destroy the whole IoT-WSN. A lot of methods are applied to discover devices that may be attacked. The energy, seizing cost, and device contribution of IoT devices are used to obtain probable attackable devices in various approaches. Optimization methods such as Grey Wolf, Dragon Fly, Cuttlefish, and Fruit Fly Optimization are also applied to enhance the selection of probable attackable IoT devices in IoT-WSNs. In this chapter, node capture attacks, optimization methods, and encryption approaches were explained and efficiency examined based on characteristics such as security, attacking rounds, energy expenditure, confusion, diffusion, and compromised traffic.

REFERENCES

1. A. K. Nuristani and J. Thakur, "Security Issues and Comparative Analysis of Security Protocols in wireless Sensor Networks: A Review", *International Journal of Computer Science and Engineering (JCSE)*, Vol. 6, Issue 10, 2018, pp. 436–444.
2. A. M. Tripathi and S. Singh, "A literature review on algorithms for the load balancing in cloud computing environments and their future trends", *Computer Modelling & New Technologies*, Vol. 21, Issue 1, 2017, pp. 64–73.
3. A. Alharbi, "Security Issues in Wireless Sensor Networks", *Indian Journal of Science and Technology*, Vol. 10, Issue 25, 2017, pp. 1–5.
4. A. Bojchevski and S. Gunnemann, "Adversarial Attacks on Node Embeddings", *cs. LG,* 2018, pp. 1–12.
5. A. Khare, R. Gupta and P. K. Shukla, "A Grey Wolf Optimization Algorithm (GWOA) For Node Capture Attack To Enhance The Security Of Wireless Sensor Network", *International Journal of Scientific & Technology Research*, Vol. 9, Issue 3, 2020, pp. 206–209.
6. A. Khare, R. Gupta and P. K. Shukla, "A Dragonfly Optimization Algorithm (DOA) for Node Capture Attack to Improve the Security of Wireless Sensor Network", *International Journal of Emerging Technology and Advanced Engineering,* Vol. 9, Issue 10, 2019, pp. 167–171.
7. A. Jain and T. Singh, "Securing Communication in IoT Ecosystem Using Cryptographic Algorithms", *International Journal of Engineering and Advanced Technology (IJEAT),* Vol. 9, Issue 1, 2019, pp. 7258–7268.
8. A. Munir and A. G. Ross, "Optimization Approaches in Wireless Sensor Networks", *Intechopen*, 2010, pp. 1–27.
9. A. Albakri, L. Harn and S. Song, "Hierarchical Key Management Scheme with Probabilistic Security in a Wireless Sensor Network (WSN)", *Security and Communication Networks, Hindawi*, 2019, pp. 1–11.
10. A. Kul, E. N. Azin, O. Ozdemir and S. Sahin, "IoT-Smart Contract Rule Based Secure Communication Scheme for Healthcare System", *Easy Chair preprints*, 2019, pp. 1–13.
11. B. Butani, P. K. Shukla and S. Silakari, "An Exhaustive Survey on Physical Node Capture Attack in WSN", *International Journal of Computer Applications*, Vol. 95, No. 3, 2014, pp. 32–39.

12. C. Xiong, S. Li, L. Liu, R. Li and Y. Jin, "A Hybrid Key Pre-distribution Scheme for Wireless Sensor Networks", *IOP Conf. Series, Journal of Physics*, 2019, pp. 1–18.

13. C. Lin and G. Wu, "Enhancing the attacking efficiency of the node capture attack in WSN: a matrix approach", *J Supercomput, Springer Science &Business Media*, 2013, pp. 1–19.

14. C. Lin, G. Wu, C. W. Yu, and L. Yao, "Maximizing destructiveness of node capture attack in wireless sensor networks", *J Supercomput, Springer Science & Business Media*, Vol. 71, 2015, pp. 3181–321.

15. C. Lin, T. Qiu, M. S. Obaidat, C. W. Yu, L. Yao and G. Wu, "MREA: a minimum resource expenditure node capture attack in wireless sensor networks", *Security And Communication Networks, Wiley Online Library*, Vol. 9, 2016, pp. 5502–5517.

16. D. Woods, M. Abdallah, S. Bagchi, S. Sundaram, and T. Cason, "Network Defense and Behavioral Biases: An Experimental Study", *National Science Foundation*, 2020, pp. 1–40.

17. D. Molina, J. Poyatos, J. D. Ser, S. Garcia, A. Hussain and F. Herrera, "Comprehensive Taxonomies of Nature- and Bio-inspired Optimization: Inspiration versus Algorithmic Behavior, Critical Analysis and Recommendations", *cs.AI*, 2020, pp. 1–76.

18. G. Padmavathi and D. Shanmugapriya, "A Survey of Attacks, Security Mechanisms and Challenges in wireless Sensor Networks", *International Journal of Computer Science and Information Security*, Vol. 4, No. 1, 2009, pp. 1–10.

19. G. Wu, X. Chen, and M. S. Obaidat, "A High Efficient Node Capture Attack Algorithm in Wireless Sensor Network based on Route Minimum Key Set", *Security and Communication Networks*, Vol. 6, 2013, pp. 230–238.

20. H. R. Shaukat, F. Hashim, M. A. Shaukat and K. A. Alezabi, "Hybrid Multi-Level Detection and Mitigation of Clone Attack s in Mobile Wireless Sensor Network (MWSN)", *Sensors*, MDPI, Vol. 20, 2020, pp. 1–23.

21. H. Chan, A. Perrig and D. Song, "Random Key Predistribution Schemes for Sensor Networks", *Bosch research*, 2003, pp. 1–17.

22. H. Yamano, K. Asatani and I. Sakata, "Evaluating Nodes of Latent Mediators in Heterogeneous Communities", *Scientific Reports in Nature Research*, 2020, pp. 1–11.

23. I. Q. Kolagar, H. H. S. Javadi, and M. Anzani, "Hypercube Bivariate-Based Key Management for Wireless Sensor Networks", *Journal of Sciences, Islamic Republic of Iran*, University of Tehran, Vol. 28, No. 3, 2017, pp. 273–285.

24. I. Butun, P. Osterberg and H. Song, "Security of the Internet of Things: Vulnerabilities, Attacks and Countermeasures", *IEEE Communications Surveys and Tutorials*, 2019, pp. 1–25.

25. J. W. Ho, "Distributed detection of Node Capture Attacks in Wireless Sensor Networks", *Intechopen*, 2010, pp. 345–363.

26. K. Chowdary, and K.V.V. Satyanarayana, "Malicious Node Detection and Reconstruction of Network In Sensor Actor Network", *Journal of Theoretical and Applied Information Technology*, Vol. 95, No.3, 2017, pp. 582–591.

27. M. R. Alshammari and K. M. Elleithy, "Efficient and Secure Key Distribution Protocol for Wireless Sensor Networks", *Sensors*, MDPI, Vol. 18, 2018, pp. 1–25.

28. M. Waniek, T. P. Michalak and A. Alshamsi, "Strategic Attack & Defense in Security Diffusion Games", *ACM Transactions on Intelligent Systems and Technology*, Vol. 11, No. 1, 2019, pp. 1–35.

29. M. J. Lagarde, "Security Assessment of Authentication and Authorization Mechanisms in Ethereum, Quorum, Hyperledger Fabric and Corda", *Ecole Polytechnique Federale De lausannne*, 2019, pp. 1–99.

30. M. Srivastava and A. Dixit, "Blackhole Detection Technique in WSN-A Review", *Technical Research Organization India*, Vol. 4, issue 8, 2017, pp. 47–55.
31. M. A. Hamid, M. M. O. Rashid and C. S. Hong, "Routing Security in Sensor Network: HELLO Flood Attack and Defense", *Next Generation Wireless Systems*, 2006, pp. 77–81.
32. M. Huang and B. Yu, "Fuzzy Guard: A DDoS attack prevention extension in software-defined wireless sensor networks", *KSII Transactions on Internet and Information Systems*, Vol. 13, No. 7, 2019, pp. 3671–3689.
33. M. Wazid, "LDAKM-EIoT: Lightweight Device Authentication and Key management Mechanism for Edge-Based IoT Deployment", *Sensors, MDPI*, Vol. 19, 2019, pp. 1–21.
34. M. Iqbal, M. Naeem, A. Anpalagan, A. Ahmed and M. Azam, "Wireless Sensor Network Optimization: Multi-Objective Paradigm", *Sensors, MDPI*, Vol. 15, 2015, pp. 1–49.
35. M. Ehdaie, N. Alexiou, M. Ahmadian, M. R. Aref and P. Papadimitratos, "Mitigating Node Capture Attack in Random Key Distribution Schemes through Key Deletion", *Journal of Communication Engineering*, Vol. 6, No. 2, 2017, pp. 1–10.
36. N. Labraoui, M. Gueroui and L. Sekhri, "On-Off Attacks Mitigation against Trust Systems in Wireless Sensor Networks", *HAL*, 2018, pp. 1–12.
37. O. Brun, Y. Yin, J. A. Gonzalez, M. Ramos and E. Gelenbe, "IoT Attack Detection with Deep Learning", *HAL*, 2019, pp. 1–11.
38. P. Senger and N. Bhardwaj, "A Survey on Security and Various Attacks in Wireless Sensor Network", *International Journal of Computer Sciences and Engineering (JCSE)*, Vol. 5, Issue 4, 2017, pp. 78–84.
39. P. Tague and R. Poovendran, "Modeling Adaptive Node Capture Attacks in Multi-hop Wireless Networks", *Ad Hoc Networks, Elsevier*, Vol. 5, 2007, pp. 801–814.
40. P. Tague, D. Slater, J. Rogers and R. Poovendran, "Evaluating the Vulnerability of Network Traffic Using Joint Security and Routing Analysis", IEEE Computer Society, 2009, pp. 111–123.
41. P. Tague and R. Poovendran, "Modeling Node Capture Attacks in Wireless Sensor Networks", *IEEE Xplore*, 2008, pp. 1–5.
42. P. K. Shukla, S. Goyal, R. Wadhvani, M. A. Rizvi, P. Sharma, and N. Tantubay, "Finding Robust Assailant Using Optimization Functions (FiRAO-PG) in Wireless Sensor Network", *Hindawi Publishing Corporation, Mathematical Problems in Engineering*, 2015, pp. 1–8.
43. P. and R. K. Chauhan, "Review on Security attacks and Countermeasures in Wireless Sensor Networks", *International Journal of Advanced Research in Computer Science*, Vol. 8, No. 5, 2017, pp. 1275–1284.
44. P. De, Y. Liu and S. K. Das, "Deployment aware Modeling of Node Compromise Spread in Wireless Sensor Networks Using Epidemic Theory", *ACM*, 2008, pp. 1–29.
45. P. Ahlawat and M. Dave, "An attack resistant key predistribution scheme for wireless sensor Networks", *Journal of King Saud University – Computer and Information Sciences, Elsevier*, 2018, pp. 1–13.
46. P. Ahlawat and M. Dave, "An attack model based highly secure key management scheme for wireless sensor Networks", *6th International Conference on Smart Computing and Communications, ICSCC, Elsevier*, Kurukshetra, India, 2017, pp. 1–7.
47. Q. Zhang and W. Zhang, "Accurate Detection of Selective Forwarding Attack in Wireless Sensor Networks", *Advances in Cyber Physical Social Systems (CPSS), International Journal of Distributed Sensor Networks*, Vol. 15, No. 1, 2019, pp. 1–8.

48. Q. Liu, J. Yin, V. C. M. Leung and Z. Cai, "FADE: Forwarding Assessment Based Detection of Collaborative Grey Hole Attacks in WMNs", *IEEE Transactions on Wireless Communications*, 2013, pp. 1–14.

49. R. D. Graaf, I. Hegazy, J. Horton and R. S. Naini, "Distributed Detection of Wormhole Attacks in Wireless Sensor Networks", *LNICST*, Vol. 28, 2010, pp. 208–223.

50. R. Bhatt, P. Maheshwary, P. Shukla, P. Shukla, M. Shrivastava and S. Changlani, "Implementation of Fruit Fly Optimization Algorithm (FFOA) to Escalate the Attacking Efficiency of Node capture Attack in Wireless Sensor Networks (WSN)", *Computer Communications, Elsevier*, Vol. 149, 2020, pp. 134–145.

51. S. Lalar, S. Bhushan and Surendar, "Exploration of Detection Method of Clone Attack in Wireless Sensor Network", *International Journal of Recent Technology and Engineering (IJRTE)*, Vol. 8, Issue 4, 2019, pp. 2440–2448.

52. S. Horawalavithana, J. A. Flores, J. Skvoretz and A. Lamnitchi, "The risk of node re-identification in labeled social graphs", *Applied Network Science, Springer*, Vol. 4, 2019, pp. 1–20.

53. S. Kumar, D. Datta and S. K. Singh, "Black Hole Algorithm and Its Application", *Computational Intelligence, Springer*, 2015, pp. 147–170.

54. S. K. Yang, Y. M. Shiue, Z. Y. Su, I. H. Liu and C. G. Liu, "An Authentication Information Exchange Scheme in WSN for IoT applications", *IEEE Access*, 2019, pp. 1–11.

55. S. Lagraa, M. Cailac, S. Rivera, F. Beck and R. State, "Real-time attack detection on robot cameras: A self-driving car application", *HAL*, 2019, pp. 1–9.

56. S. Hong, S. Lim and J. Song, "Unified Modelling Language based Analysis of Security Attacks in Wireless Sensor Networks: A Survey", *KSII Transactions on Internet and Information System*, Vol. 5, No. 4, 2011, pp. 805–821.

57. S. Hong and S. Lim, "Analysis of attack Models via Unified Modeling Language in Wireless Sensor Networks: A Survey Study", *IEEE*, 2010, pp. 692–696.

58. W. du, J. Deng, Y. S. Han, and P. K. Varshney, "A Key Pre-distribution Scheme for Sensor Networks Using Deployment Knowledge", *IEEE INFOCOM*, 2004, pp. 586–597.

59. W. Li, B. Li, Y. Zhao, P. Wang and F. Wei, "Cryptanalysis and Security Enhancement of Three Authentication Schemes in Wireless Sensor Networks", *Hindawi Wireless Communications and Mobile Computing*, 2018, pp. 1–12.

60. Z. Wang, C. Zhou and Y. Liu, "Efficient Hybrid Detection of Node Replication Attacks in Mobile Sensor Networks", *Mobile Information Systems, Hindawi*, 2017, pp. 1–13.

3 Internet of Everything-Based Advanced Big Data Journey for the Medical Industry

Piyush Gupta,[1] Bhupendra Verma,[2] and Mahesh Pawar[1]
[1] Rajiv Gandhi Technical University,
Bhopal, Madhya Pradesh, India
[2] Technocrats Group of Institutions, Bhopal,
Madhya Pradesh, India

CONTENTS

3.1 INTRODUCTION

IoT (Internet of Things) is a combination of various communication devices and smart electronics that sense and communicate with each other [1]. In recent years, IoT devices brought a revolution in the field of biomedical applications by looking at

DOI: 10.1201/9781003145035-3

several challenges and complications faced in the past [2]. These IoT devices can generate a significant amount of bio-medical data and also play a vital role in the development of existing automatic medical-data collection systems. When IoT devices are integrated with advanced ML (Machine Learning) algorithms, big data is essential for improvising these health systems in diagnosis, decision making as well as treatment. IoT in biomedical applications has developed research areas in applications of IoE (Internet of Everything) such as symptomatic treatments (symptomatic treatment, supportive care, supportive therapy, or palliative treatment is any medical therapy of a disease that only affects its symptoms, not the underlying cause), observation of patients as well as monitoring [3].

Generally, IoE brings together the process, people, data, and things by interconnecting them through the Internet. It influences people's lives, business, and also their industrial processes. Further, real-time information collected from multiple sensors is interconnected and implemented in people-oriented automatic processes (for example, mart city environments, smart supply chains and fitness bands) [4]. Additionally, IoE helps to accomplish environmental sustainability and socioeconomic goals as well. IoE is utilized in fossil fuel mining, remote monitoring, e-learning, automation, traffic controls, smart grids, etc. There is an enormous amount of data generated by sensors that are implanted in physical objects in specific environments. As generating and monitoring information is a constant process, keeping these devices connected to the Internet is essential to ensure uninterrupted data updates to servers.

Figure 3.1 shows the key features of IoE in hospital environments. An example of the use of the IoE is that patients with diabetes will be given ID cards, which will be scanned and linked to the cloud that stores the EHRs (Electronic Health Records) and essential laboratory results, prescriptions, and records of medical history. Nurses and physicians can access these records on computers or tablets for easy patient care.

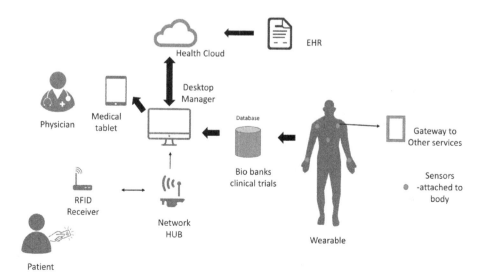

FIGURE 3.1   Revolutionary features of IoE in a hospital environment [5].

The implementation of EHRs has brought a significant change in the field of healthcare sectors. Managing the hospital records by ink-paper systems will be replaced to digital systems. The conventional ink-paper system has various limitations and it also can be missed at times. EHRs provide all the essential information in one place and also facilitate sharing this information among doctors and other healthcare providers. EHRs can optimize healthcare and even save lives. However, one huge drawback in implanting IoE is communication. Even though diverse devices possess various sensors for collecting data and information, they cannot communicate to the data center. Further, each manufacturer has its own protocols and not all sensors can communicate with each other.

Big data analytics is a predominant technology particularly in digital transformations, the integration of digital technology into all areas of a business, fundamentally changing how you operate and deliver value to customer. Further, big data has impacted on different sectors such as healthcare, geospatial communication systems, sensor networks, mobile applications, and E-commerce in a short period of time, also the rate of data arrival will be in EB (Exabytes). Due to the heterogeneous nature of healthcare sectors, apart from being massive and distinct, the high-speed data arrival becomes a highly challenging task in big data analysis. Moreover, the data of patients are present in numerous forms starting from the origin of disease followed by medical history, pre- and post-treatment process, duration of treatment, diagnostic and postoperative data such as EEG, MRI reports, X-rays, ultrasound reports, and CT scans. Big data analysis on these sectors due to its multi-dimensional methods and techniques, made it a perfect solutions for healthcare sectors. By using this advanced technology, healthcare systems become easier to access and are more cost effective.

3.2 DIMENSIONS OF BIG DATA

Big data is obtained by several websites such as Twitter, Facebook and LinkedIn. Other sources of big data are blog sites and diverse instruments such as sensors for different applications. This big data needs a new architecture, various techniques, complex algorithms as well as powerful analytics for managing high-scale data and in order to extract useful information by applying complex algorithms. As the magnitude of data exceeds a specific point, the qualitative problems become more essential than the quantitative problems in data capturing, data storing, data processing, analysis of data, as well as data visualization. Moreover, big data has several characteristics such as volatility, viscosity, virality, value, visualization, and variability.

Variety: Big data collects a variety of data from sources such as EHRs, ECGs, and sensor data for various applications, audio, social websites, and digital photos.

Velocity: Big data calculates the speed of data that is coming from different sources like sensors, machines, mobile phones, and networks. Also the data flow is constant, and incorporates unstructured and structured data formats.

Visualization: collected data must be represented in an understandable manner, and since there are various characteristics such as velocity, volume, etc., this becomes more challenging. Thus, visualization measures aim to provide a complete and clean picture of the data.

Volatility: refers to speed, through which the data moves across networks. Besides data, time also plays a major role in data analytics.

3.3 APPLICATIONS OF MEDICAL BIG DATA

The following are the applications of big data in healthcare.

* Big data and medical imaging
* Telemedicine
* Predictive analytics in healthcare sectors
* Big data could cure cancer
* Informed strategic planning by utilizing health data
* Enhancing the patient engagement
* Real-time alerting
* EHRs (Electronic Health Records)
* Patient prediction

3.4 PATIENT PREDICTION

Big data is helpful for identifying patients with complex medical histories, suffering from multiple conditions and also for indentifying the need for improved staffing. Several researchers have discussed using big data in predicting patients, in which data from different sources was integrated to predict daily and hourly patients expected to visit hospitals. Further, data scientists have used time series analysis using hospital's admission records. This has helped in predicting patient admission rates as well as rate of staff availability, thus improving the performance of staff [7]. Additionally, various ML algorithms can be used for analysis and prediction of admissions trends for future patients. When prediction is performed, correspondingly more staff can be scheduled thereby reducing waiting times of patients and also improving patient care.

3.5 ELECTRONIC HEALTH RECORDS

EHRs store patient reports like lab test results, medical histories, and demographics digitally [8]. Moreover, a secured information system (a formal, sociotechnical, organizational system designed to collect, process, store, and distribute information.) has been employed for making these EHRs available for private and public sector. Since all records are digitized data duplication is minimized so, there is much less need for paper documents.

In addition to that, EHRs can generate remainders for tracking prescriptions and scheduling lab tests.

One study suggested that in the United States a system named Health-Connect has been implemented, which was easy to share and utilize data [9]. One report from McKinsey on integrated systems on big data revolution in US healthcare indicted that approximately one million dollars have been saved due to the reduction of office visits and pathology tests for cardiovascular disease.

3.6 REAL-TIME ALERTING

By utilizing big data, real-time alerting provide a predominant features to healthcare analytics to analyze healthcare data and report unexpected or abnormal conditions to a clinician or doctor. Generally, in hospitals, real-time CDS (Clinical Decision Support) systems helps health practitioners with prescriptions and advice on spot. However, these real-time systems are costly and many health practitioners prefer their patients to stay away from hospitals unless absolutely necessary. In recent years, personal analytics have been used in the form of wearable devices such as smart watches to share medical information with healthcare providers via the cloud [10]. For instance, if there is a rapid increase in blood pressure of a particular patient the provider could receive an alert so that corresponding actions could be taken. Moreover, in the Asthmapolis system, the inhaler has GPS access, used for finding asthma trends at individual level in huge population. These data can be aggregated from CDS, thus resulting in better treatment plans for patients suffering from asthma.

3.7 ENHANCING PATIENT ENGAGEMENT

As people become more and more health conscious smart devices for monitoring pulse rate, blood pressure, sleep, and activity are becoming more common. These devices help health providers and patients identify health risks. Also, specific health trends can be identified, thus enhancing patient engagement and provider care, and further resulting in a significant reduction in the number of number of hospital visits.

3.8 INFORMED STRATEGIC PLANNING BY UTILIZING HEALTH DATA

In today's world, strategic planning in healthcare sectors is very essential, which can be provided by big data analytics. In one study an application was introduced by Google Maps for illustrating different real-time problems. Things such as the spread of any chronic disease or population growth can be represented in the form of heat maps [12].

3.9 BIG DATA COULD CURE CANCER

A system called Cancer Moonshoot has been developed to cure cancer. Academics compared this data with the availability of medical services in most heated areas and decisions could be taken with respect to healthcare strategies. This system provides treatment plans. These treatment records are mapped in order to interact with the cancer proteins, so the treatment can be planed [13]. This results in obtaining better outcomes. This also sometimes gives surprising results such as, presence of desipramine, which cures lung cancer.

Additionally, this research requires interconnecting different hospitals, institutions as well as non-profit organizations from which treatment records are available. The samples of cancer tissues of trial patients are sequenced genetically and added to worldwide cancer databases. Nevertheless, one challenge of big data analytics is incompatible data across different databases preventing access to these records.

3.10   PREDICTIVE ANALYTICS IN HEALTHCARE SECTORS

In recent years, predictive analytics has been exploited for business applications. A recent research project in the United States has gathered datasets from thirty million people, from which the study observed a good quality of delivery care [9].

Predictive analytics can help health practitioners and doctors make decisions on the basis of available datasets for better patient care. Moreover, it can be used to predict heart disease, high blood pressure as well as diabetes and guide patients on dietary plans or weight management programs [14].

3.11   TELEMEDICINE

For more than 40 years, telemedicine has been in industries that are rapidly evolving to provide increased access to high-quality healthcare that is efficient and cost-effective by the use of various technology such as smartphones, wireless devices, online VC (video conferences), and wearable devices. It provide access to health assessment, diagnosis, intervention, consultation, supervision and information across distance for medical professionals, healthcare education, and monitoring of remote patients Further, tele-surgery, another kind of remote medical service, has been performed by utilizing skilled robots with high speed and precision using real-time data from remote location as illustrated in Figure 3.2. With the help of tele-medicine, admission costs in hospitals are significantly reduced, and QoS (Quality of Service) is increased.

3.12   BIG DATA AND MEDICAL IMAGING

Big data has major contribution in Medical imaging, so, several radiologists individually can investigate every medical image, analyse them and store them for many years that will be accessed by the healthcare sectors. However, this method consumes more time and cost.

Carestream, a medical imaging provider, uses algorithms to analyse images and find specific patterns to determine diagnosis and thereby help doctors in treating diseases.

3.13   CHALLENGES OF BIG DATA IN THE MEDICAL INDUSTRY

The challenges in healthcare sectors are due to a range of numerous diseases and their critical conditions, different results, variety of treatments, analytical techniques as well as collection of several methodologies. Further, in healthcare sectors, there are various sources of big data such as biometric data, web data, medical-images,

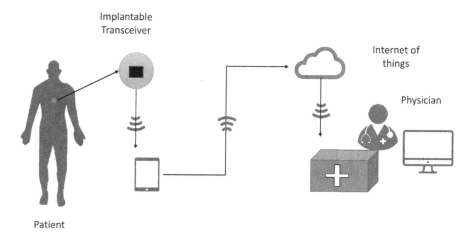

FIGURE 3.2   Remote patient monitoring [15].

reports of outpatients, electronic records, clinical data and case records. Combining these information sources generates massive datasets. Several studies have addressed the characteristics of big data in medical field and compared with traditional medical epidemiological information [16]. However, collecting these large volumes of data requires several protocols, and since this process uses costly instruments and well-trained professionals, So, it is expensive. Moreover, it is prone to various uncertainties like coding errors, missing values as well as measurement fails. The typical features of the medical big data is continuously in changes with respect to time and patient characteristics and due to this treatment and decisions may become difficult.

3.14 MISSING VALUES

Big data analytics in the healthcare sector manages the data that are collected from various sources for many purposes. However it suffers from missing variables as well as incompleteness in the datasets. The easiest way to handle the missing values is to add data values or remove case from datasets. In addition, several data mining algorithms are capable of handling missing values while pre-processing. Missing data represents various relations with the prevailing unobserved and observed data values, which are depicted as follows:

- **NMAR (Not missing at random)**: missing data is related to unobserved data.
- **MAR (Missing at random)**: missing data is not related to the unobserved data, but is related to observed data.
- **MCAR (Missing completely at random)**: missing data is not related to the unobserved and observed data. Here, the missing data would not impact the analysis process. Moreover, Stata, SAS, R, and WinBUGS are some automatic tools for handling the missing values. If the missing values are below 10%, these tools provide similar outcomes. Whereas, if the missing values are more

than 60%, the tools will fail to provide appropriate outcomes. However, the tools may provide other suggestions for the missing values between 10 and 60%.

3.15 CHALLENGES IN MEDICAL BIG DATA

Even though big data analytics has huge potential in various fields, particularly medical fields, there are certain challenges for implementing big data analytics in healthcare sectors. Since big data is a recent technology, its practical advantages are less evident [17]. Also, big data suffers from inherent methodological problems such as heterogeneity, timeliness, privacy, data incompleteness, data inconsistency, data quality, legal issues, analytical issues, instability as well as limitations in observational studies. Moreover, the quality of data must be updated, particularly in EHRs, as it is sensitive. Thus, dramatic changes are needed for solving technical issues for acquiring better outcomes. Finally, the big data analytics and clinical integration can provide several benefits, however it takes at least few years to obtain the expected integration and outcomes. Additionally, big data analytics provides efficient, improvised patient care as well as quicker response[18].

3.16 CASE STUDY OF A DIABETIC PATIENT

This chapter presents a case study on utilizing IoE in combination with big data in healthcare. By combining these two technologies, data from different patients can be easily collected and securely stored using diverse IoT nodes, and can provide performs real-time monitoring of patients.

Diabetic patients must monitor activity and diet as well blood sugar levels. Medical care of these patients is more essential, but is very challenging as there are several checks performed in a single day. The primary objective of Ref. [10] is to enable the doctors to real-time monitor the patients with diabetes. This system initially reads all the data from the sensor and then uses it to determine whether the parameters are normal by comparing the user-defined thresholds with healthcare measures. Further, this device calculates the average value of each medical measure and communicates this to MongoBD. Figure 3.3 demonstrates this real-world monitoring of blood pressure.

Moreover, the study evaluated the efficiency of the suggested system by performing experimental analysis with cluster, formed by three nodes, which is powered by Intel i7 processor with 3.4GHz and 16GB ram. For evaluating scalability, the study used an open source EHR generator like Box 1 for producing the medical data.

3.17 SUMMARY

Health is considered a global challenge for humankind. According to the World Health Organization, constant patient monitoring is said to be the highest standard in hospitals. Big data plays a vital role in patient care by monitoring patients' vital signs and keeping EHRs up to date and maintained across different platforms. Moreover,

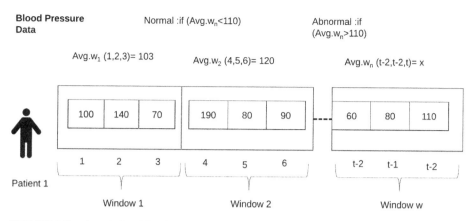

FIGURE 3.3 A real-time blood pressure monitoring system [10].

big data analytics is used for capturing and analysing patient data to determine diagnosis and the best treatment plans using the most current data.

REFERENCES

[1] M. Javaid and A. Haleem, "Industry 4.0 applications in medical field: a brief review," *Current Medicine Research and Practice,* vol. 9, pp. 102–109, 2019.

[2] A. Chandy, "A review on IoT based medical imaging technology for healthcare applications," *Journal of Innovative Image Processing (JIIP),* vol. 1, pp. 51–60, 2019.

[3] M. A. Khan, M. T. Quasim, N. S. Alghamdi, and M. Y. Khan, "A secure framework for authentication and encryption using improved ECC for IoT-based medical sensor data," *IEEE Access,* vol. 8, pp. 52018–52027, 2020.

[4] J. S. Raj and S. Jennifer, "Optimized Mobile Edge Computing Framework for IoT based Medical Sensor Network Nodes," *Journal of Ubiquitous Computing and Communication Technologies (UCCT),* vol. 3, pp. 33–42, 2021.

[5] D. V. Dimitrov, "Medical internet of things and big data in healthcare," *Healthcare informatics research,* vol. 22, pp. 156–163, 2016.

[6] R. Kashyap, "Applications of wireless sensor networks in healthcare," in *IoT and WSN Applications for Modern Agricultural Advancements: Emerging Research and Opportunities*, ed: IGI Global, 2020, pp. 8–40.

[7] F. Abdali-Mohammadi, M. N. Meqdad, and S. Kadry, "Development of an IoT-based and cloud-based disease prediction and diagnosis system for healthcare using machine learning algorithms," *IAES International Journal of Artificial Intelligence,* vol. 9, p. 766, 2020.

[8] F. Khennou, Y. I. Khamlichi, and N. E. H. Chaoui, "Improving the use of big data analytics within electronic health records: a case study based OpenEHR," *Procedia Computer Science,* vol. 127, pp. 60–68, 2018.

[9] H. S. Jim, A. I. Hoogland, N. C. Brownstein, A. Barata, A. P. Dicker, H. Knoop, *et al.,* "Innovations in research and clinical care using patient-generated health data," *CA: a cancer journal for clinicians,* vol. 70, pp. 182–199, 2020.

[10] L. Benhlima, "Big data management for healthcare systems: architecture, requirements, and implementation," *Advances in bioinformatics,* vol. 2018, 2018.

[11] A. E. Sharma, N. A. Rivadeneira, J. Barr-Walker, R. J. Stern, A. K. Johnson, and U. Sarkar, "Patient engagement in health care safety: an overview of mixed-quality evidence," *Health affairs,* vol. 37, pp. 1813–1820, 2018.

[12] M. Hasan, M. Shahjalal, M. Z. Chowdhury, and Y. M. Jang, "Real-time healthcare data transmission for remote patient monitoring in patch-based hybrid OCC/BLE networks," *Sensors,* vol. 19, p. 1208, 2019.

[13] W. J. Hopp, J. Li, and G. Wang, "Big data and the precision medicine revolution," *Production and Operations Management,* vol. 27, pp. 1647–1664, 2018.

[14] S. Kumar and M. Singh, "Big data analytics for healthcare industry: impact, applications, and tools," *Big data mining and analytics,* vol. 2, pp. 48–57, 2018.

[15] "slideshare.net/hsplmkting/webinar-iot-in-healthcare-an-overview."

[16] N. Mehta and A. Pandit, "Concurrence of big data analytics and healthcare: A systematic review," *International journal of medical informatics,* vol. 114, pp. 57–65, 2018.

[17] R. Kashyap and A. D. Piersson, "Big data challenges and solutions in the medical industries," in *Handbook of Research on Pattern Engineering System Development for Big Data Analytics,* ed: IGI Global, 2018, pp. 1–24.

[18] S. Shilo, H. Rossman, and E. Segal, "Axes of a revolution: challenges and promises of big data in healthcare," *Nature medicine,* vol. 26, pp. 29–38, 2020.

4 IoT in Smart Rehabilitation

Meena Gupta, Ruchika Kalra, and Prakash Kumar
Amity University, Noida, UP, India

CONTENTS

4.1 INTRODUCTION

In today's world there are numerous conditions that are entering countries and creating a great impact on healthcare; as medical conditions are progressing so are the management techniques.[1] Rehabilitation is a field where it is essential that the patient is well placed, where smart rehabilitation occurs and acts smartly and efficiently towards the patient.[2] Here this smart rehabilitation requires a team to be efficient, from various fields of healthcare, to provide complete care. Smart rehabilitation is a wide term which includes small integrated and separate technologies to come together and work individually depending upon the technology behind it.[3] The patient and healthcare workers require a working platform in which the medical team and patient are aware of health progressing, allowing the communication system to be a helping hand. IoT systems, E-health, tele health, mobile health and EKSO bionics are involved in this kind of system as smart rehabilitation.[4]

Smart rehabilitation is working on the architecture-based system where there is the basic combination of three components that are motion sensor, server for communication and the station handling all the base.[5] This connects the machine to human

DOI: 10.1201/9781003145035-4

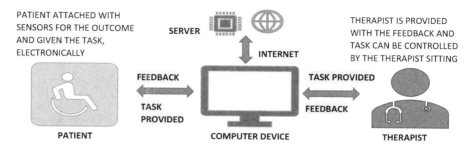

FIGURE 4.1   Structure of a smart rehabilitation system.

with different sensors allowing the part of the human body to be rehabilitated with the control of the task calculated and provided by the therapist according to the requirement and the feedback and monitoring is done smartly by the sensors attached, this progression is presented in the biofeedback manner and shared with all the health team whether present or not present at the time of the rehabilitation[6,7] (see Figure 4.1).

4.2   SENSORS BEHIND SMART REHABILITATION SYSTEMS

Here the system consists of the sensors which are applied on the affected arm/ limb, which includes accelerometers, magnetic sensors and gyroscopes that are inertial sensors which allows all the rotation motion, velocity at different angles to be recorded and allowed to work.[8] The base station allows the patient to have the personal device such as computer screen. The movement created is recorded as the data and feedback in all the directions which is formed and shared through a major server acting as the messenger to the therapist, allowing the record maintenance and feedback of the patient progression and the range accomplished in various degrees of freedom[9,10] (see Figure 4.2). The sensors attached in the rehabilitation system specially for the athletic sports person works on each variant of changes that are recorded at the time of rehabilitation, such as the physiological changes of the level of muscle activity,[11,12] the consumption of the lactose, muscle degeneration and regeneration, requirement of the glucose accordingly.[13] The requirement of the oxygen is measured according to the level of the fatigue present as the task and assessment is done accordingly, such as the posture correction, gait correction and the muscle enhancement for the better results with efficiency.[14]

Advanced sensors are utilized in the various medical applications from patient to athlete, where muscle control to ergonomics to consumption of the food and other physiological requirements are recorded.[15] Sensors are placed from head to toe to analyze each muscle action and correction to be created and the effort initiated.[16] From ECG to measurement of the variation of the urine infection is determined with the help of the sensors.[17] The rehabilitation is decided from the data collected and recorded in the computer device to form the personal record which is directly shared to the therapist involved and rehabilitation team involved beside.[18] The sensors provide the feedback to the patient too, which improves the effort of the patient and allows them to work positively.[19,20]

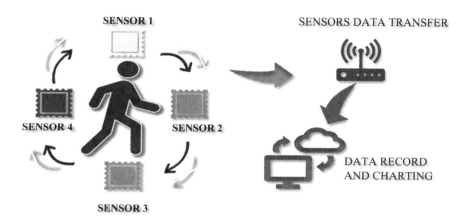

FIGURE 4.2 Sensors in a working system.

4.3 BIO MICROELECTRONIC MECHANICAL SYSTEMS (MEMS)[21]

Microelectronic mechanical systems are micro-fabricated devices structured from circuits that are integrated allowing all the function to be possible with electrical too. The micro-fabrication is done in layers with quite a long process. These small devices are really helpful in the healthcare system too which can be implanted in the human body as bio sensors which are used in smart rehabilitation as part of internet device.[22,23] These devices can be inside the human body measuring fluid analysis, pH, blood pressure.[24,25] Nowadays there are stents used in angioplasty of main arteries supplying brain and heart that are blocked, these devices prevent the stenosis and provide the ballooning in the arteries.[26,27] Other Bio MEMS can provide the immune-isolation benefits and drug delivery systems where the implants that are fitted in the human body transfuses the drug after a duration of time when the timing of the dosage and quantity is set for the particular time[28,29] (see Figure 4.3). There are cardiac pacemakers, devices implanted in the human body with complete success and efficiency to create the electric stimulation to the heart to achieve the complete circulation and prevent fibrillation and arrhythmias.[30,31] These MEMS are the small devices which keeps track in very precise manner in millimeter to nanometer in every measure for which it is implanted. The pitch for the upcoming enhancement of Bio MEMS is so on peak that in upcoming days it will be able to replace all the human body parts or augment them.[32,33]

4.4 INTERNET OF THINGS IN REHABILITATION

Nowadays, technology has increased in every profession from learning to rules creation, from structure build to other fields, but it is also required in and has entered the healthcare society.[34] Earlier, the technology was only in the medical set up without a link between each other to share but the Internet-of-Things has allowed for this task with the help of internet sharing from each device to recording and presentation

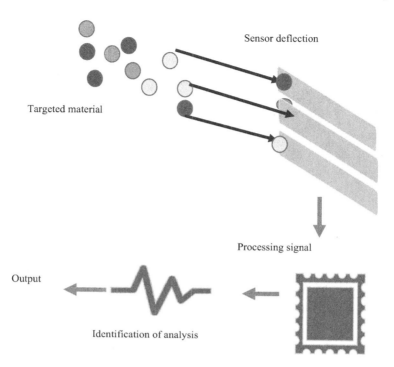

FIGURE 4.3   Bio MEMS working.

devices, creating an ease in the data arrangement and sharing.[35] The data is highly informative which cannot be minutely shared from one device to another but the technology of IoT in healthcare allows the transfer from device to machine, from sensor to screen.[36] This has made the medical record to be more easily detectable and accurately diagnosed. This technology is not limited to the healthcare system but also to rehabilitation systems which have turned the atmosphere of the improvement to the next level due to precision in charting the progression in the rehabilitation.[37] IoT-based systems not only ease the progression but are also reliable in keeping secret sensitive data, such as the medical record.[38] The precision present in this technology tends to minimize the human error and can be an improvement in the error correction when it comes to terms of life and death.[39] Now the technology of the IoT in healthcare has increased to the framework to include cloud storage which provides an advantage that the data can be viewed by any healthcare worker and be secured in every aspect[40] (see Figure 4.4). This provides an advantage to the patient and the family as the data is shared with patient and family to be more clear, as nowadays the education level had allowed the upcoming requirement of the clearness of the patient progression or deterioration and treatment and management that is provided for them.[41] The infrastructure behind IoT stands with five components starting from sensor technology, intelligent network, cloud computing, analyzing the biological data and a smart organization to handle this.[42] The IoT system is so efficient to use

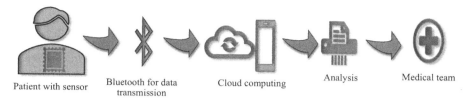

Patient with sensor   Bluetooth for data   Cloud computing   Analysis   Medical team
                       transmission

FIGURE 4.4   Internet of Things in rehabilitation.

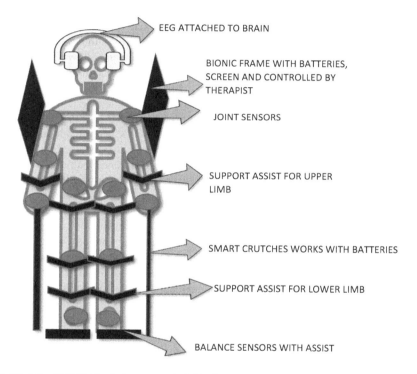

EEG ATTACHED TO BRAIN

BIONIC FRAME WITH BATTERIES,
SCREEN AND CONTROLLED BY
THERAPIST

JOINT SENSORS

SUPPORT ASSIST FOR UPPER
LIMB

SMART CRUTCHES WORKS WITH BATTERIES

SUPPORT ASSIST FOR LOWER LIMB

BALANCE SENSORS WITH ASSIST

FIGURE 4.5   EKSO bionic in smart rehabilitation.

that nowadays this complete system is arranged so that homes can be turned into smart homes, so that every plus and minus of the patient is recorded and data is exchanged with the doctors so as to turn the home into a safe and successful place for rehabilitation after the surgeries and treatment plan followed at home.[43]

4.5 EKSO BIONICS IN REHABILITATION

There are various exoskeletons that are very successful in gait rehabilitation where massive neurological problems come up, the EKSO bionic is one of the exoskeletons which comes under the title of robotic smart rehabilitation[44] (see Figure 4.5). This is a frame covering the whole body with multiple sensors and the server is attached on the back of the patient allowing motion to be controlled by the therapist through the sensors. The artificial limbs in the frames walk in the same way as normal limbs and allow for the muscle action to be in the same direction of the damaged muscle and make the gait healthy with complete support. The sensors are working from head to toe to facilitate the movement, allowing the movement to be successful and healthy.[45,46] The procedure is created to help with the damage that is created at the spinal cord injury level and the loss that is created, this alters the EMG level of the functioning muscle of the upper limb and lower limb and spinal muscles;[47] the exoskeleton not only works for the lower limb but also for the complete body structure so as to create the functional movement.[48,49] The algorithm works so that the powered exoskeleton works on the physical impairment to be solved, this is controlled with the battery powered control with the help of sensors and joysticks transferring the data to the computer interface and allowing the charting for the impairment above.[50] On the other hand there are brain-machine interfaces where the sensors work for the sensation capabilities, cognitive capabilities inside the patient's brain, capability behind the patient's brain and structuring the physiological changes inside the brain that are recorded on the side of the brain and restructuring the physical changes that are required in the powered skeleton and changing and allowing the result to be more efficient.[51] This brain-machine interface can be viewed through invasive or non-invasive means that are recorded on the electroencephalogram and allow the patient to be completely encircled with sensors at the brain level so as to create an effective powered exoskeleton.[52] There are exoskeletons of different varieties and different approach such as Lokomat, EKSO bionics and so on.[53] The EKSO bionic is created such that it is a complete powered frame with bilateral support such as a cane or walker beside,[54] this makes the bilateral fixation of the lower limb allowing the limb to be supported for the balance.[55] Due to its large and bulky structure the concern comes that how can the weak neurological patient hold the frame, but the inertia present in the structure of machine creates no weight on the patient's body,[56] in addition, it carries the weight of the patient so as to bear weight on the lower limb progressively, according to the charting of the limb muscles present at the EMG of every muscle, creating a feedback to the patient and therapist and altering the functioning of the machine side by side.[57] The machine works step by step, at first controlled by the therapist then, after understanding the exoskeleton, the patient is himself settled to control with the external button beside and, after so many days of usage the machine is just controlled by the muscle action of the hip allowing to walk forward.[58] The progression is done on the basis of the EMG enhancement of the muscle activation and physiological changes occurring both at the brain-machine interface, EMG and EEG arriving.[59] The analysis report is created on every muscle action, synergy, reaction and the sensation changes occurring at the dermatological level as well as the brain levels.[60,61]

4.6   MOBILE HEALTH

Mobile health, as the term defines, is creating a usage of mobile devices for health purposes as, nowadays, the mobile is the device carried by almost every person and, in general' is easily operated, so the thought of using a mobile device for health purposes turns out to be useful.[62] The basic, initial usage of the mobile device was for calling, messaging and using search engines on the internet but the technology has improved so well that it has allowed for many applications that act as the source for useful medical applications, such as heart monitoring, ECG monitoring, steps as per requirement of the body, fluid consumption as per required dietary advice.[63,64] The Internet of Things in healthcare has facilitated mobile healthcare and has facilitated the beginning of mobile health in the smart rehabilitation.[65] The technology changed from wired to non-wired and the internet allowed the layers to set in between and be a part of the communication for data transfer.[66] The precision is now such that the technology that used to be invasive is turning out to be less invasive in nature now that it can be measured with the help of the sensors placed in smartphones.[67] The ECG, temperature and pulse rate were variables that were measured with the different devices, but the mobile device has made it easier to utilize the same.[68] Mobile health with IoT systems were installed with the intelligent systems that not only provides you the reading but also the security measures are completely taken care of for the same, such as the process for the safety and privacy issues.[69] The technology is not only limited to mobile devices that the sensors are placed in but also to external sensor devices that are applied to body segments, such as a heart monitor that is kept near the pocket of the shirt to measure the ECG and heart rate of the patient (the sensor presents, with precision, data that is shared to the mobile device of the patient just with wireless communication and shared with the rehabilitation team).[70] Similarly, the device worn around the feet calculates the steps taken and acts as the pedometer allowing the count of the steps to be used for motivation. The sensors for the wireless connections are either controlled by the Bluetooth, WiFi or Infrared technology and communicate with the mobile device and health worker.[71] Mobile health is upcoming and can be an easier method to create the medical data and safety but is expensive and, with patient doubt for precision of the results, relies on further treatment and management.[72,73]

4.7 TELEHEALTH

Telehealth is the technology where numerous healthcare sectors are covered with the help of tele-communication, where medicine and assistance towards rehabilitation is provided.[74,75] Previously, the data was difficult to be carried out and saved but the Internet of Things technology has allowed for more precise storage within cloud computing[76] and greater reliability and accessibility for every person who is linked in for his or her medical treatment.[77] The network earlier followed by the telehealth was not that reliable or accessible for the medical team, but IoT systems allowed the network to, with the presence of the reliability and feature of cloud computing, create analysis reports more securely and cheaply, improving access and keeping it up to date.[78] The IoT system links the sensors gathering the readings of the patient and stores within cloud computing,[79] creating the charts and further leading to access directly to the medical team allowing steps to be initiated with the help of the telehealth and making sure that the patient is healthy and safe.[80] The hard work for computing for telehealth has decreased with the addition of the IoT system, allowing minimum errors and maximum results reliability.[81] This reliable feature allows normal homes to be smart homes and the sense of satisfaction to the patient that he or she is still in observation of the medical team and being treated well.[82]

4.8   E-HEALTH

This term defines the management and review of health through electronic media, whether this be through mobile health or the different devices that are related to other communication devices.[83,84] The device is connected through various sensors, with the help of the Internet of Things, as a system working virtually and robotically towards patient rehabilitation.[85] Electronic health provides a platform for a medical facility that was earlier only possible in person, but technology improvement has led to the development of communication technology, which is enhanced with the help of internet facilities available at patient homes.[86,87] The internet allows a decrease in hospital stay and a betterment in the medical facility and assessment of the patient through various sensors, such as diabetic sensors, blood pressure sensors and heart monitoring, and even acceptance of changes occurring at the nervous system level allowing a direct link even if the patient is far from a doctor and from a hospital setting.[88] This allows the E-health to monitor and assist with patient rehabilitation. The technology had increased the precision in communication, helping in the healthcare society and promoting confidence in the medical team and patient setting.[89] This allows a patient to be satisfied while at home rather than in the hospital setting.[90] The IoT-based E-health system is a three-layer structure, from getting the data from the sensor layer to cloud computing and analyzing at the cloud layer, and then the third layer transfers the data to patients and the doctor's desk.[91,92]

4.9   BRAIN-COMPUTER INTERFACE[93]

This section discusses a technology that can connect the patient to the environment without the patient speaking,[94] where the patient's brain signals provide a connection between the brain and computer enabling communication graphs to allow a communicative state, using machines such as prosthesis to follow commands accordingly[95] (see Figure 4.6). This technology leads to an interaction of the brain with objects attached to the person at three different levels: scalp, cortical and brain.[96] It leads to communication between the person and machine without the patient saying anything, rather it uses analysis and decoding of the readings obtained from sensors present at the brain level.[97] The most utilized signals are electric signals as used in the post synaptic membrane where the polarity changes according the activation of the ion gated channels or specific voltage channels.[98] The BCI can be either invasive or non-invasive depending upon the nature of determination required.[99,100] The less invasive, that at scalp level, provides the information superficially and takes time to determine the decoding and delay in the communication and is generally used just prior to the surgery such as in case of epileptic changes occurring.[101] Whereas the invasive sensors, that are kept at the cortex or sub-dural level, provides immediate response with more accuracy[102] (see Figure 4.7). There are types of non-invasive types where the BCI-based EEG is the best for interpretation and the invasive can be involving surgery and implantation of the device at the level of requirement. These devices are highly useful for the patients with neurodegenerative disorder where the neuro muscular disorder patient does not

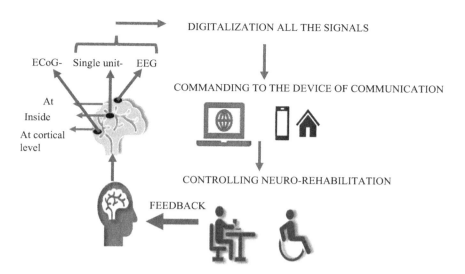

FIGURE 4.6 Brain-computer interface.

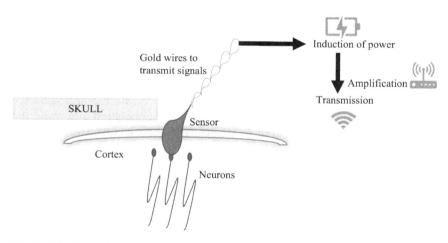

FIGURE 4.7 Recording of brain signals.

have the voluntary control over the muscular system; this device has a large positive role in neuro rehabilitation.[103]

Brain-computer interface depicts the inner thoughts of the person to act as the commands for himself.[104] The interface is not the depiction of person's muscle, tendons, not the electro-encephalogram as they are just the graphical distribution which cannot be understood.[105] The neuro-rehabilitation has been taken to the next level which allows direct interface with the central nervous system allowing the peripheral nervous system to act accordingly.[106] This brain-computer interface is not the mind reader but leads the mind to work rather than muscles.[107] The device encodes the brain activity and decodes the intentional process of the task to accomplish. There are four basic step processes, first is acquisition of the signal to extraction of the signals to translation and in the end of the output that is the command to be followed.[108] The acquisition of signals involves the measuring of the brain signals which are then amplified and processed in the computer system.[109] The extraction of features involves the analyses of what is represented into the output where the graphical presentation translation produces the output commands and the correlation should be relevant. The responses gathered from the brain activity are either transient or oscillatory in nature.[110] BCI systems at present are triggered by time, as in corticography or encephalography. Translation process occurs so as to change the output to relevant commands, but priorly ensure, while providing translation, that it has to be spontaneous in nature so as to provide the dynamic nature of use and covers all the functional translation to the device so as to act according to patient.[111] The output of the device is suggested to be the loop closer where the movement of the prosthesis is observed and all the functions are performed according to actions and feedback created in the patient's mindset.[112]

4.10   FUTURE CHALLENGES

The IoT-based system is upcoming in the world of smart rehabilitation, which has changed the valuation of the health sector.[113] The advantage of smart rehabilitation has enabled health to be near the doorstep and more accessible to the patient, with all-time availability of the patient whenever required.[114] This has not only allowed the patient to be followed but also the normal person to be attentive towards health and motivated in how to improve their health and have a more active lifestyle.[115]

The challenges behind smart rehabilitation are to create the accessibility of the technology behind the Internet of Things to the population and make them understand the usage behind and replicate the parameters involved and how to use it.[116,117] Smart rehabilitation is within reach in developed countries but lags way behind in the under developed and developing countries where the smartphones are not the daily requirement of the person.[118] The other challenge is that it is easy to depict and create the level of reliability on the patient and their family but difficult to make them understand, as still the thinking is that, to be more reliable, the patient has to approach the medical team and be present on every observation as the physical contact creates, with the patient and doctor, more confidence on the patient treatment decision than relying on the E health measure.[119,120] The challenge is also to keep the profile and the data secured but there are some applications that do not allow for the same as the cyber crime is one of the increasing and the cyber security is one of the costliest securities so as to keep the medical records in the safe place.[121,122]

4.11   DISCUSSION

The study refers to technology changing the lives not only in improving the life easiness in work, study and other day-to-day needs but also improving the healthcare system which is allowing it to be more realistic with upcoming challenges that has to be faced by the engineers, patient and health workers to be better by this idea.[123] The smart rehabilitation system links every cross connection and makes it secure while having the exchange of the information.[124]

According to the studies, smart rehabilitation does not state that only the patient can be accessed but also the normal person who wants an active lifestyle can also be one of them. Applications that are under the technology of Internet of Things allow for handy assessment, such as a fit-bit present on the wrist which allows the measuring of the active life cycle, that a person is having and a chart to depict not only one day but all over the analysis that not only give a result physical but also a hit on psychological aspects and make the patient want to be on the healthier side.[125,126] The studies depicting the increase in the technology in sensors have allowed health workers and patients to be comfortable and at ease in life anywhere, not necessary to be near doctor or medical staff.[127] The sensor is all over, covering the head to toe, coming with every physical, physiological, psychological and records of every activity with progression and data analysis.[128,129] The smart rehabilitation systems have allowed for the healthy system in pandemic, allowing people to be healthy and less in contact with the hospital environment.[130] The IoT has allowed a spectrum for health care in wide aspect with keeping the environment of hospitality and observation at home and limit the effect of the hospital exposure.[131,132] The E-health, tele health and mobile health are the hands of the smart rehabilitation system under the term of Internet of Things of smart rehabilitation system which provides the features of health services in hands.[133]

4.12 CONCLUSION

Internet of Things for smart rehabilitation is an upcoming technology for the population dependent on the technology system for their daily needs. The technology has improved the measure for health care and taken it to the next level, by keeping health system conveniently handy by use of a hand set. This smart rehabilitation system can come up with new chapters after day-to-day research and development by meeting the challenges and overcoming them.

REFERENCES

1 de Sousa TB, Rocha IF, Loiola FS, da Conceição GR, de Souza CG, Ruwer SG. Application of the Internet of Things in the healthcare field. In 2nd International Symposium on Supply Chain 4.0 2018 (p. 16).
2 Sathya M, Madhan S, Jayanthi K. Internet of things (IoT)-based health monitoring system and challenges. International Journal of Engineering & Technology. 2018;7(1.7):175–8.
3 Mohapatra S, Kumar A, Mohapatra S. From a literature review to a conceptual framework for affordable quality healthcare service using internet of things (IOT) network. International Journal of Enterprise Network Management. 2018;9(1):11–21.
4 Jeong JS, Han O, You YY. A design characteristics of smart healthcare system as the IoT application. Indian Journal of Science and Technology. 2016 Oct;9(37):1–8.
5 Zheng H, Davies R, Stone T, Wilson S, Hammerton J, Mawson SJ, Ware PM, Black ND, Harris ND, Eccleston C, Hu H. SMART rehabilitation: implementation of ICT platform to support home-based stroke rehabilitation. In International Conference on Universal Access in Human-Computer Interaction 2007 Jul 22 (pp. 831–840). Springer, Berlin, Heidelberg.

6   Zheng H, Davies R, Zhou H, Hammerton J, Mawson SJ, Ware PM, Black ND, Eccleston C, Hu H, Stone T, Mountain GA. SMART project: application of emerging information and communication technology to home-based rehabilitation for stroke patients. International Journal on Disability and Human Development. 2006 Jul 1;5(3):271.

7   Ware P, Hammerton J, Mawson SJ, Mountain GA, Zheng H, Davies RJ, BLACK N, Harris ND, Wilson S, T STONE CE, Hu H. SMART: Developing information and communication technology for self management of stroke and chronic conditions. at home. In 21st International Symposium on Human Factors in Telecommunication 2008 Mar.

8   Zheng H, Davies RJ, Black ND. Web-based monitoring system for home-based rehabilitation with stroke patients. In 18th IEEE Symposium on Computer-Based Medical Systems (CBMS'05) 2005 Jun 23 (pp. 419–424). IEEE.

9   Mountain GA, Ware PM, Hammerton J, Mawson SJ, Zheng H, Davies R, Black N, Zhou H, Hu H, Harris N, Eccleston C. The SMART project: a user led approach to developing applications for domiciliary stroke rehabilitation. In Designing accessible technology 2006 (pp. 135–144). Springer, London.

10 Zhou H, Hu H. Inertial motion tracking of human arm movements in stroke rehabilitation. In IEEE International Conference Mechatronics and Automation, 2005 2005 Jul 29 (Vol. 3, pp. 1306–1311). IEEE.

11 Allen H, Coggan AR, McGregor S. Training and racing with a power meter. VeloPress; 2019 Apr 22.

12 Siirtola P, Laurinen P, Röning J, Kinnunen H. Efficient accelerometer-based swimming exercise tracking. In 2011 IEEE Symposium on Computational Intelligence and Data Mining (CIDM) 2011 Apr 11 (pp. 156–161). IEEE.

13 Ishido H, Takahashi H, Nakai A, Takahata T, Matsumoto K, Shimoyama I. 6-Axis force/torque sensor for spike pins of sports shoes. In 2015 28th IEEE International Conference on Micro Electro Mechanical Systems (MEMS) 2015 Jan 18 (pp. 257–260). IEEE.

14 Zagatto AM, Beck WR, Gobatto CA. Validity of the running anaerobic sprint test for assessing anaerobic power and predicting short-distance performances. The Journal of Strength & Conditioning Research. 2009 Sep 1;23(6):1820–7.

15 Camomilla V, Bergamini E, Fantozzi S, Vannozzi G. Trends supporting the in-field use of wearable inertial sensors for sport performance evaluation: A systematic review. Sensors. 2018 Mar;18(3):873.

16 Eskofier BM, Lee SI, Baron M, Simon A, Martindale CF, Gaßner H, Klucken J. An overview of smart shoes in the internet of health things: gait and mobility assessment in health promotion and disease monitoring. Applied Sciences. 2017 Oct;7(10):986.

17 Mancini A, Frontoni E, Zingaretti P. Mechatronic system to help visually impaired users during walking and running. IEEE transactions on intelligent transportation systems. 2018 Jan 10;19(2):649–60.

18 Barkallah E, Freulard J, Otis MJ, Ngomo S, Ayena JC, Desrosiers C. Wearable devices for classification of inadequate posture at work using neural networks. Sensors. 2017 Sep;17(9):2003.

19 Hoettinger H, Mally F, Sabo A. Activity recognition in surfing-a comparative study between hidden markov model and support vector machine. Procedia engineering. 2016 Jan 1;147:912–7.

20 Zhang B, Jiang S, Wei D, Marschollek M, Zhang W. State of the art in gait analysis using wearable sensors for healthcare applications. In 2012 IEEE/ACIS 11th International Conference on Computer and Information Science 2012 May 30 (pp. 213–218). IEEE.

21 Kovacs, G. T., Maluf, N. I., & Petersen, K. E. (1998). Bulk micromachining of silicon. Proceedings of the IEEE, 86(8), 1536–1551.

22 Service, R. F. (2002). Can sensors make a home in the body? Science, 297(5583), 962–3.

23 Abel, P. U., & von Woedtke, T. (2002). Biosensors for in vivo glucose measurement: can we cross the experimental stage. Biosensors and Bioelectronics, 17(11–12), 1059–1070.

24 Gough, D. A., & Armour, J. C. (1995). Development of the implantable glucose sensor: What are the prospects and why is it taking so long? Diabetes, 44(9), 1005–1009.

25 Meyerhoff, M. E. (1993). In vivo blood-gas and electrolyte sensors: Progress and challenges. TrAC Trends in Analytical Chemistry, 12(6), 257–266.

26 Wirthlin, D. J., Alcocer, F., Whitley, D., & Jordan Jr, W. D. (2002). Use of hybrid aortic stent grafts for endovascular repair of abdominal aortic aneurysms: Indications and outcomes. Journal of Surgical Research, 108(1), 14–19.

27 Hiatt, B. L., Ikeno, F., Yeung, A. C., & Carter, A. J. (2002). Drug-eluting stents for the prevention of restenosis: In quest for the holy grail. Catheterization and cardiovascular interventions, 55(3), 409–417.

28 Desai, T. A., Hansford, D. J., Kulinsky, L., Nashat, A. H., Rasi, G., Tu, J., ... & Ferrari, M. (1999). Nanopore technology for biomedical applications. Biomedical Microdevices, 2(1), 11–40.

29 Ahmed, A., Bonner, C., & Desai, T. A. (2001). Bioadhesive microdevices for drug delivery: a feasibility study. Biomedical Microdevices, 3(2), 89–96.

30 Hayes, D. L. (1999). Evolving indications for permanent pacing. The American Journal of Cardiology, 83(5), 161–165.

31 Werner, J., Meine, M., Hoeland, K., Hexamer, M., & Kloppe, A. (2000). Sensor and control technology for cardiac pacing. Transactions of the Institute of Measurement and Control, 22(4), 289–302.

32 Santini, Jr, J. T., Richards, A. C., Scheidt, R., Cima, M. J., & Langer, R. (2000). Microchips as controlled drug-delivery devices. Angewandte Chemie International Edition, 39(14), 2396–2407.

33 Grayson, A. C. R., Shawgo, R. S., Johnson, A. M., Flynn, N. T., Li, Y., Cima, M. J., & Langer, R. (2004). A BioMEMS review: MEMS technology for physiologically integrated devices. Proceedings of the IEEE, 92(1), 6–21.

34 Kumar N. IoT architecture and system design for healthcare systems. In2017 International Conference on Smart Technologies for Smart Nation (SmartTechCon) 2017 Aug 17 (pp. 1118–1123). IEEE.

35 Onasanya A, Elshakankiri M. Smart integrated IoT healthcare system for cancer care. Wireless Networks. 2019 Jan 2:1–6.

36 Ge SY, Chun SM, Kim HS, Park JT. Design and implementation of interoperable IoT healthcare system based on international standards. In2016 13th IEEE annual consumer communications & networking conference (CCNC) 2016 Jan 9 (pp. 119–124). IEEE.

37 Darshan KR, Anandakumar KR. A comprehensive review on usage of Internet of Things (IoT) in healthcare system. In2015 International Conference on Emerging Research in Electronics, Computer Science and Technology (ICERECT) 2015 Dec 17 (pp. 132–136). IEEE.

38 Aceto G, Persico V, Pescapé A. The role of Information and Communication Technologies in healthcare: taxonomies, perspectives, and challenges. Journal of Network and Computer Applications. 2018 Apr 1;107:125–54.

39 Catherwood PA, Steele D, Little M, McComb S, McLaughlin J. A community-based IoT personalized wireless healthcare solution trial. IEEE journal of translational engineering in health and medicine. 2018 May 8;6:1–3.

40 Tyagi S, Agarwal A, Maheshwari P. A conceptual framework for IoT-based healthcare system using cloud computing. In2016 6th International Conference-Cloud System and Big Data Engineering (Confluence) 2016 Jan 14 (pp. 503–507). IEEE.

41 Gupta PK, Maharaj BT, Malekian R. A novel and secure IoT-based cloud centric architecture to perform predictive analysis of users activities in sustainable health centres. Multimedia Tools and Applications. 2017 Sep 1;76(18):18489–512.

42 Jeong JS, Han O, You YY. A design characteristics of smart healthcare system as the IoT application. Indian Journal of Science and Technology. 2016 Oct;9(37):1–8.

43 Rodic Trmcic B, Labus A, Radenkovic B. Internet of Things in ehealth: application of wearables for stress management. In XV International Symposium SymOrg 2016 2016 (pp. 387–395).

44 Tefertiller C, Pharo B, Evans N, Winchester P. Efficacy of rehabilitation robotics for walking training in neurological disorders: A review. Journal of Rehabilitation Research & Development. 2011 Jul 1;48(4).

45 Benito-Penalva J, Edwards DJ, Opisso E, Cortes M, Lopez-Blazquez R, Murillo N, Costa U, Tormos JM, Vidal-Samsó J, Valls-Solé J, Medina J. Gait training in human spinal cord injury using electromechanical systems: effect of device type and patient characteristics. Archives of physical medicine and rehabilitation. 2012 Mar 1;93(3):404–12.

46 Goffredo M, Iacovelli C, Russo E, Pournajaf S, Di Blasi C, Galafate D, Pellicciari L, Agosti M, Filoni S, Aprile I, Franceschini M. Stroke Gait Rehabilitation: A Comparison of End-Effector, Overground Exoskeleton, and Conventional Gait Training. Applied Sciences. 2019 Jan;9(13):2627.

47 Sale P, Russo EF, Scarton A, Calabrò RS, Masiero S, Filoni S. Training for mobility with exoskeleton robot in spinal cord injury patients: A pilot study. Eur. J. Phys. Rehabil. Med. 2018 Oct 1;54:745–51.

48 Chang SH, Afzal T, Berliner J, Francisco GE. Exoskeleton-assisted gait training to improve gait in individuals with spinal cord injury: a pilot randomized study. Pilot and feasibility studies. 2018 Dec;4(1):1–0.

49 Nam KY, Kim HJ, Kwon BS, Park JW, Lee HJ, Yoo A. Robot-assisted gait training (Lokomat) improves walking function and activity in people with spinal cord injury: a systematic review. Journal of neuroengineering and rehabilitation. 2017 Dec 1;14(1):24.

50 Stevenson AJ, Mrachacz-Kersting N, van Asseldonk E, Turner DL, Spaich EG. Spinal plasticity in robot-mediated therapy for the lower limbs. Journal of neuroengineering and rehabilitation. 2015 Dec;12(1):1–7.

51 Louie DR, Eng JJ, Lam T. Gait speed using powered robotic exoskeletons after spinal cord injury: a systematic review and correlational study. Journal of neuroengineering and rehabilitation. 2015 Dec 1;12(1):82.

52 Dobkin B, Apple D, Barbeau H, Basso M, Behrman A, Deforge D, Ditunno J, Dudley G, Elashoff R, Fugate L, Harkema S. Weight-supported treadmill vs over-ground training for walking after acute incomplete SCI. Neurology. 2006 Feb 28;66(4):484–93.

53 Alcobendas-Maestro M, Esclarín-Ruz A, Casado-López RM, Muñoz-González A, Pérez-Mateos G, González-Valdizán E, Martín JL. Lokomat robotic-assisted versus overground training within 3 to 6 months of incomplete spinal cord lesion: randomized controlled trial. Neurorehabilitation and neural repair. 2012 Nov;26(9):1058–63.

54 Swinnen E, Duerinck S, Baeyens JP, Meeusen R, Kerckhofs E. Effectiveness of robot-assisted gait training in persons with spinal cord injury: a systematic review. Journal of rehabilitation medicine. 2010 Jun 5;42(6):520–6

55 Palermo AE, Maher JL, Baunsgaard CB, Nash MS. Clinician-focused overview of bionic exoskeleton use after spinal cord injury. Topics in spinal cord injury rehabilitation. 2017 Jun;23(3):234–44.

56 Landau ID, Lozano R, M'Saad M, Karimi A. Adaptive control: algorithms, analysis and applications. Springer Science & Business Media; 2011 Jun 6.

57 Moreno JC, Barroso F, Farina D, Gizzi L, Santos C, Molinari M, Pons JL. Effects of robotic guidance on the coordination of locomotion. Journal of neuroengineering and rehabilitation. 2013 Dec 1;10(1):79.

58 Jin X, Cai Y, Prado A, Agrawal SK. Effects of exoskeleton weight and inertia on human walking. In 2017 IEEE International Conference on Robotics and Automation (ICRA) 2017 May 29 (pp. 1772–1777). IEEE.

59 Moreno JC, Barroso F, Farina D, Gizzi L, Santos C, Molinari M, Pons JL. Effects of robotic guidance on the coordination of locomotion. Journal of neuroengineering and rehabilitation. 2013 Dec 1;10(1):79.

60 Swank C, Wang-Price S, Gao F, Almutairi S. Walking with a robotic exoskeleton does not mimic natural gait: a within-subjects study. JMIR rehabilitation and assistive technologies. 2019;6(1):e11023.

61 De Luca A, Bellitto A, Mandraccia S, Marchesi G, Pellegrino L, Coscia M, Leoncini C, Rossi L, Gamba S, Massone A, Casadio M. Exoskeleton for Gait Rehabilitation: Effects of Assistance, Mechanical Structure, and Walking Aids on Muscle Activations. Applied Sciences. 2019 Jan;9(14):2868.

62 Jara AJ, Zamora MA, Skarmeta AF. Knowledge acquisition and management architecture for mobile and personal health environments based on the internet of things. In 2012 IEEE 11th International Conference on Trust, Security and Privacy in Computing and Communications 2012 Jun 25 (pp. 1811–1818). IEEE.

63 Atzori L, Iera A, Morabito G. The internet of things: A survey. Computer networks. 2010 Oct 28;54(15):2787–805.

64 Giusto D, Iera A, Morabito G, Atzori L, editors. The internet of things: 20th Tyrrhenian workshop on digital communications. Springer Science & Business Media; 2010 Mar 10.

65 Kan C, Chen Y, Leonelli F, Yang H. Mobile sensing and network analytics for realizing smart automated systems towards health internet of things. In 2015 IEEE International Conference on Automation Science and Engineering (CASE) 2015 Aug 24 (pp. 1072–1077). IEEE.

66 Istepanian RS, Hu S, Philip NY, Sungoor A. The potential of Internet of m-health Things "m-IoT" for non-invasive glucose level sensing. In 2011 Annual International Conference of the IEEE Engineering in Medicine and Biology Society 2011 Aug 30 (pp. 5264–5266). IEEE.

67 Lymberis A. Smart wearables for remote health monitoring, from prevention to rehabilitation: current R&D, future challenges. In 4th International IEEE EMBS Special Topic Conference on Information Technology Applications in Biomedicine, 2003. 2003 Apr 24 (pp. 272–275). IEEE.

68 Sharif S, Mobin I, Mohammed N. Augmented quick health. International Journal of Computer Applications. 2016 Jan;134(11):1–6.

69 Islam SR, Kwak D, Kabir MH, Hossain M, Kwak KS. The internet of things for health care: a comprehensive survey. IEEE access. 2015 Jun 1;3:678–708.

70 Hengstler S. Wireless Health: Making Your Devices Talk A Review, Solution, and Outlook for Wireless Health Connectivity.

71 Habbal M. Bluetooth low energy–assessment within a competing wireless world. In Proceedings of the Wireless Congress 2012.

72 Shaltis PA, Reisner A, Asada HH. Wearable, cuff-less PPG-based blood pressure monitor with novel height sensor. In 2006 International Conference of the IEEE Engineering in Medicine and Biology Society 2006 Aug 30 (pp. 908–911). IEEE.

73 K. J. Cho and H. H. Asada, "Wireless, battery-less stethoscope for wearable health monitoring," in Bioengineering Conference, 2002. Proceedings of the IEEE 28th Annual Northeast, 2002, pp. 187–188.

74 Rolim CO, Koch FL, Westphall CB, Werner J, Fracalossi A, Salvador GS. A cloud computing solution for patient's data collection in health care institutions. In2010 Second International Conference on eHealth, Telemedicine, and Social Medicine 2010 Feb 10 (pp. 95–99). IEEE.

75 Al-Qurishi M, Al-Rakhami M, Al-Qershi F, Hassan MM, Alamri A, Khan HU, Xiang Y. A framework for cloud-based healthcare services to monitor noncommunicable diseases patient. International journal of distributed Sensor Networks. 2015 Mar 5;11(3):985629.

76 Gachet D, de Buenaga M, Aparicio F, Padrón V. Integrating internet of things and cloud computing for health services provisioning: The virtual cloud carer project. In 2012 Sixth International Conference on Innovative Mobile and Internet Services in Ubiquitous Computing 2012 Jul 4 (pp. 918–921). IEEE.

77 Doukas C, Maglogiannis I. Bringing IoT and cloud computing towards pervasive healthcare. In 2012 Sixth International Conference on Innovative Mobile and Internet Services in Ubiquitous Computing 2012 Jul 4 (pp. 922–926). IEEE.

78 Forkan A, Khalil I, Tari Z. CoCaMAAL: A cloud-oriented context-aware middleware in ambient assisted living. Future Generation Computer Systems. 2014 Jun 1;35:114–27.

79 Xu B, Xu L, Cai H, Jiang L, Luo Y, Gu Y. The design of an m-Health monitoring system based on a cloud computing platform. Enterprise Information Systems. 2017 Jan 2;11(1):17–36.

80 Zamil MG. A verifiable framework for smart sensory systems. International Journal of Embedded Systems. 2017;9(5):413–25.

81 Rahmani AM, Gia TN, Negash B, Anzanpour A, Azimi I, Jiang M, Liljeberg P. Exploiting smart e-Health gateways at the edge of healthcare Internet-of-Things: A fog computing approach. Future Generation Computer Systems. 2018 Jan 1;78:641–58.

82 Al Zamil MG, Samarah SM, Rawashdeh M, Hossain MA. An ODT-based abstraction for mining closed sequential temporal patterns in IoT-cloud smart homes. Cluster Computing. 2017 Jun 1;20(2):1815–29.

83 D'Ambrogio A, Gaudio P, Gelfusa M, Luglio M, Malizia A, Roseti C, Zampognaro F, Giglio A, Pieroni A, Marsella S. Use of integrated technologies for fire monitoring and first alert. In 2016 IEEE 10th International Conference on Application of Information and Communication Technologies (AICT) 2016 Oct 12 (pp. 1–5). IEEE.

84 Rojas I, Ortuño F, editors. Bioinformatics and Biomedical Engineering: 5th International Work-Conference, IWBBIO 2017, Granada, Spain, April 26–28, 2017, Proceedings. Springer; 2017 Apr 7.

85 Scarpato N, Pieroni A, Di Nunzio L, Fallucchi F. E-health-IoT universe: A review. management. 2017;21(44):46.

86 Ennafiri M, Mazri T. Internet of Things for Smart Healthcare: a Review on a Potential Iot Based System and Technologies to Control COVID-19 Pandemic. The International Archives of Photogrammetry, Remote Sensing and Spatial Information Sciences. 2020;44:219–25.

87 Ennafiri M, Mazri T. Internet of Things for Smart Healthcare: a Review on a Potential Iot Based System and Technologies to Control COVID-19 Pandemic. The International Archives of Photogrammetry, Remote Sensing and Spatial Information Sciences. 2020;44:219–25.

88 Urbanczyk T, Peter L. Database development for the urgent department of hospital based on tagged entity storage following the IoT concept. IFAC-Papers. 2016 Jan 1;49(25):278–83.

89 Alex G, Varghese B, Jose JG, Abraham A. A modern health care system using IoT and Android. Int. J. Comput. Sci. Eng., IJCSE. 2016 Apr;8(4).

90 Andreu Y, Chiarugi F, Colantonio S, Giannakakis G, Giorgi D, Henriquez P, Kazantzaki E, Manousos D, Marias K, Matuszewski BJ, Pascali MA. Wize Mirror-a smart, multisensory cardio-metabolic risk monitoring system. Computer Vision and Image Understanding. 2016 Jul 1;148:3–22.

91 e Sá JO, Sá JC, Sá CC, Monteiro M, Pereira JL. Baby steps in E-Health: Internet of Things in a doctor's office. In World Conference on Information Systems and Technologies 2017 Apr 11 (pp. 909–916). Springer, Cham.

92 Rahimi Moosavi S, Nguyen Gia T, Rahmani AM, Nigussie E, Virtanen S, Isoaho J, Tenhunen H. SEA: a secure and efficient authentication and authorization architecture for IoT-based healthcare using smart gateways. In Procedia Computer Science 2015 (Vol. 52, pp. 452–459). Elsevier.

93 Wolpaw, J., & Wolpaw, E. W. (Eds.). (2012). Brain-computer interfaces: principles and practice. OUP USA.

94 Wolpaw, J. R., & Wolpaw, E. W. (2012). Brain-computer interfaces: something new under the sun. Brain-computer interfaces: principles and practice, 14.

95 Wolpaw, J. R., McFarland, D. J., & Vaughan, T. M. (2000). Brain-computer interface research at the Wadsworth Center. IEEE Transactions on Rehabilitation Engineering, 8(2), 222–226.

96 Wolpaw, J. R., Birbaumer, N., McFarland, D. J., Pfurtscheller, G., & Vaughan, T. M. (2002). Brain-computer interfaces for communication and control. Clinical neurophysiology: official journal of the International Federation of Clinical Neurophysiology, 113(6), 767–791.

97 Wickelgren, I. (2003). Tapping the mind. Science, 299(5606), 496–499.

98 Berger, H. (1929). Über das elektroenkephalogramm des menschen. Archiv für psychiatrie und nervenkrankheiten, 87(1), 527–570.

99 Krusienski, D. J., & Shih, J. J. (2011). Control of a visual keyboard using an electrocorticographic brain–computer interface. Neurorehabilitation and neural repair, 25(4), 323–331.

100 Krusienski, D. J., & Shih, J. J. (2011). Control of a brain–computer interface using stereotactic depth electrodes in and adjacent to the hippocampus. Journal of neural engineering, 8(2), 025006.

101 Akhtari, M., Bryant, H. C., Mamelak, A. M., Heller, L., Shih, J. J., Mandelkern, M., ... & Sutherling, W. W. (2000). Conductivities of three-layer human skull. Brain Topography, 13(1), 29–42.

102 Hochberg, L. R., Serruya, M. D., Friehs, G. M., Mukand, J. A., Saleh, M., Caplan, A. H., ... & Donoghue, J. P. (2006). Neuronal ensemble control of prosthetic devices by a human with tetraplegia. Nature, 442(7099), 164–171.

103 Junwei, L., Ramkumar, S., Emayavaramban, G., Thilagaraj, M., Muneeswaran, V., Rajasekaran, M. P., ... & Hussein, A. F. (2018). Brain computer interface for neurodegenerative person using electroencephalogram. IEEE Access, 7, 2439–2452.

104 Pfurtscheller, G., Neuper, C., Guger, C., Harkam, W. A. H. W., Ramoser, H., Schlogl, A., ... & Pregenzer, M. A. P. M. (2000). Current trends in Graz brain-computer interface (BCI) research. IEEE transactions on rehabilitation engineering, 8(2), 216–219.

105 Kennedy, P. R., Bakay, R. A., Moore, M. M., Adams, K., & Goldwaithe, J. (2000). Direct control of a computer from the human central nervous system. IEEE Transactions on rehabilitation engineering, 8(2), 198–202.

106 Birbaumer, N., & Cohen, L. G. (2007). Brain–computer interfaces: communication and restoration of movement in paralysis. The Journal of physiology, 579(3), 621–636.

107 Tan, D., & Nijholt, A. (2010). Brain-computer interfaces and human-computer interaction. In Brain-Computer Interfaces (pp. 3–19). Springer, London.

108 Wolpaw, J. R., Birbaumer, N., McFarland, D. J., Pfurtscheller, G., & Vaughan, T. M. (2002). Brain–computer interfaces for communication and control. Clinical Neurophysiology, 113(6), 767–791.

109 Vaid, S., Singh, P., & Kaur, C. (2015, February). EEG signal analysis for BCI interface: A review. In 2015 fifth international conference on advanced computing & communication technologies (pp. 143–147). IEEE.

110 McFarland, D. J., Anderson, C. W., Muller, K. R., Schlogl, A., & Krusienski, D. J. (2006). BCI meeting 2005-workshop on BCI signal processing: feature extraction and translation. IEEE transactions on neural systems and rehabilitation engineering, 14(2), 135–138.

111 McFarland, D. J., Anderson, C. W., Muller, K. R., Schlogl, A., & Krusienski, D. J. (2006). BCI meeting 2005-workshop on BCI signal processing: feature extraction and translation. IEEE transactions on neural systems and rehabilitation engineering, 14(2), 135–138.

112 Pfurtscheller, G., Allison, B. Z., Bauernfeind, G., Brunner, C., Solis Escalante, T., Scherer, R., ... & Birbaumer, N. (2010). The hybrid BCI. Frontiers in neuroscience, 4, 3.

113 Shahid N, Aneja S. Internet of Things: Vision, application areas and research challenges. In2017 International Conference on I-SMAC (IoT in Social, Mobile, Analytics and Cloud)(I-SMAC) 2017 Feb 10 (pp. 583–587). IEEE.

114 Zhong RY, Ge W. Internet of things enabled manufacturing: a review. International Journal of Agile Systems and Management. 2018;11(2):126–54.

115 Kodali RK, Swamy G, Lakshmi B. An implementation of IoT for healthcare. In2015 IEEE Recent Advances in Intelligent Computational Systems (RAICS) 2015 Dec 10 (pp. 411–416). IEEE.

116 Baker SB, Xiang W, Atkinson I. Internet of things for smart healthcare: Technologies, challenges, and opportunities. IEEE Access. 2017 Nov 29;5:26521–44.

117 Pawar AB, Ghumbre S. A survey on IoT applications, security challenges and counter measures. In2016 International Conference on Computing, Analytics and Security Trends (CAST) 2016 Dec 19 (pp. 294–299). IEEE.

118 Farahani B, Firouzi F, Chang V, Badaroglu M, Constant N, Mankodiya K. Towards fog-driven IoT eHealth: Promises and challenges of IoT in medicine and healthcare. Future Generation Computer Systems. 2018 Jan 1;78:659–76.

119 Nižetić S, Šolić P, González-de DL, Patrono L. Internet of Things (IoT): Opportunities, issues and challenges towards a smart and sustainable future. Journal of Cleaner Production. 2020 Nov 20;274:122877.

120 Reddy ON, Sivaiah BV, Kumar BN. Health Iot. Smart Health using Iot. 2020, 11(4).

121 Strielkina A, Illiashenko O, Zhydenko M, Uzun D. Cybersecurity of healthcare IoT-based systems: Regulation and case-oriented assessment. In 2018 IEEE 9th International Conference on Dependable Systems, Services and Technologies (DESSERT) 2018 May 24 (pp. 67–73). IEEE.

122 Strielkina A, Kharchenko V, Uzun D. Availability models for healthcare IoT systems: Classification and research considering attacks on vulnerabilities. In 2018 IEEE 9th International Conference on Dependable Systems, Services and Technologies (DESSERT) 2018 May 24 (pp. 58–62). IEEE.

123 Fan YJ, Yin YH, Da Xu L, Zeng Y, Wu F. IoT-based smart rehabilitation system. IEEE transactions on industrial informatics. 2014 Jan 24;10(2):1568–77.

124 Baker SB, Xiang W, Atkinson I. Internet of things for smart healthcare: Technologies, challenges, and opportunities. IEEE Access. 2017 Nov 29;5:26521–44.

125 Ullah K, Shah MA, Zhang S. Effective ways to use Internet of Things in the field of medical and smart health care. In 2016 International Conference on Intelligent Systems Engineering (ICISE) 2016 Jan 15 (pp. 372–379). IEEE.

126 Islam SR, Kwak D, Kabir MH, Hossain M, Kwak KS. The internet of things for health care: a comprehensive survey. IEEE access. 2015 Jun 1;3:678–708.

127 Singh B, Bhattacharya S, Chowdhary CL, Jat DS. A review on internet of things and its applications in healthcare. Journal of Chemical and Pharmaceutical Sciences. 2017 Jan;10(1):447–52.

128 Kanase P, Gaikwad S. Smart hospitals using internet of things (iot). International Research Journal of Engineering and Technology (IRJET). 2016 Mar;3(03).

129 García L, Parra L, Jimenez JM, Lloret J, Lorenz P. IoT-Based Smart Irrigation Systems: An Overview on the Recent Trends on Sensors and IoT Systems for Irrigation in Precision Agriculture. Sensors. 2020 Jan;20(4):1042.

130 Nolin J, Olson N. The internet of things and convenience. Internet Res.. 2016 Feb;26(2):360–76.

131 Singh P. Internet of things based health monitoring system: opportunities and challenges. International journal of advanced research in computer Science. 2018;9(1).

132 Bhatt Y, Bhatt C. Internet of things in healthcare. In Internet of things and big data technologies for next generation HealthCare 2017 (pp. 13–33). Springer, Cham.

133 Rahmani AM, Gia TN, Negash B, Anzanpour A, Azimi I, Jiang M, Liljeberg P. Exploiting smart e-Health gateways at the edge of healthcare Internet-of-Things: A fog computing approach. Future Generation Computer Systems. 2018 Jan 1;78:641–58.

5 Internet of Things in Smart and Intelligent Healthcare Systems

Puja Gupta, Mukul Shukla, Neeraj Arya, and Upendra Singh
Shri Govindram Seksaria Institute of Technology and
Science, Indore, Madhya Pradesh, India

CONTENTS

5.1   INTRODUCTION

There are many electrical gadgets on the market now that feature IoT systems. Many of them are present in common electronic devices such as smart watch, IP cameras, smart band, cellphones, home entertainment systems, and children's toys, but they are also present in automobile parts, medical equipment, and domestic appliances. These are generally equipped with the requisite intelligence of IoT systems. The chances of these being deployed are so high that IoT systems and their significance have made their way into the fields of cybernetics and information technology. IoT Systems are defined by the System Technology Platform as a mix of hardware and software incorporated in a single unit for a designated job to operate an external process via the internet communication channel. It has an electronic module with a microprocessor and other programmable electronics control devices, which are put in the system and may be controlled remotely over the internet. IoT systems are designed to work even when there is no human-machine connection, and they can respond to events in real time and from anywhere on the planet. Not only do personal computers communicate with the environment mouse, keypad, I/O, and graphical interface, but sensors, activators, and special transmission medium between wired and wireless communications all work in concert to operate things on a global scale.

As the number of old and lone senior citizens grows, necessary medical facilities would almost certainly require additional technology contributions in the near future. Important health supervision policies will be delegated to ambient systems with secure and reliable wireless connection among IoT-based healthcare systems and supervising authorities. Implanted medical devices, remote isolated implanted rehabilitative technologies and healthcare services provide prevention of serious illness, patients' irregular pressure on chronic disease, first-aid treatment, and excellent care.

Due to advancements in diagnosis and therapy, such as fine diagnostics, preventative medical examinations, robot assisted treatment, and medication efficiency, hospital stays are becoming increasingly brief. In other words, these medical centers are treating an increasing number of individuals. They spend the most of their time at home rather than in hospitals. This strategy is more persuasive psychologically and also provides a fair cost and the capacity for patients to be healthy and comfortable at home. The majority of these individuals live alone, and they are the intended audience for monitoring health systems that provide online form verification and real-time monitoring of health issues. Telemedicine systems have exploded in popularity over the years. Numerous, they offer a range of sensor attachments and monitoring mechanisms. Health supervisory systems must contain a critical characteristic of an unnamed intelligent healthcare-based IoT system that can provide anamnesis regarding patients' and medical facilities' health check statuses in real time. Participants may at any time verify their illness and fitness status and share it with their doctors and observer.

The sensors that measure the biological signals of the item serve as the link in between diagnostic person and man. This is a very different sort of measurement from what is performed in a hospital biochemical laboratory. The measuring signal may simply educate us in real time about current and historical bio signal patterns. During the rehabilitative phase, time spent in home care might result in a twenty-four-hour study of cardiac output, sleep cycles, and so on. When data from on-body and stationary sensors are combined, the signal entropy on a person's health condition rises. As stated, bio signals will be transmitted to modular integrated medical sensor parameter detectors, and important parameters will be extracted using a sophisticated signal processing approach (see Figure 5.1).

To check one's health, an artificial proposed system with a training skill set is used to process an efficient signal conditioning mechanism. The practitioner has genuine knowledge of the patient's health situation and can refer them to a doctor if their condition becomes such that this is unavoidable.

5.2 LITERATURE SURVEY

We conducted a review prior to presenting a new healthcare platform. The research's objective was to get an understanding of the existing status and potential developments in IoT-based smart healthcare. The research of "IoT" was exhaustive and included an

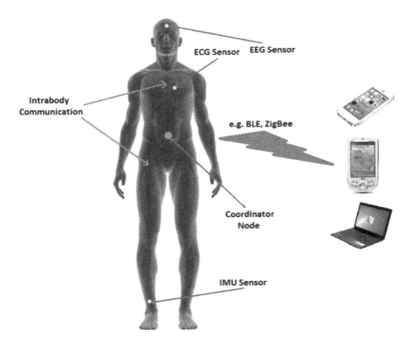

ECG Sensor   EEG Sensor

Intrabody
Communication

e.g. BLE, ZigBee

Coordinator
Node

IMU Sensor

FIGURE 5.1   Protocol for body area wireless networks [12].

analysis of relationships and limits. The primary objective of the "Internet of Things" is to guarantee that, when used in conjunction with "electronic sensor" gadgets, World Wide Web (WWW) technology and mobile transmission and reception are commonly accessible. Real-time remote monitoring helps supervision of patients from outside traditional clinical settings (e.g. at home), hence increasing access to human service offices while decreasing costs [1].

The pulse oximeter, heartbeat, respiration, muscle activity, temperature, oxygen levels, hypertension, motion, glucose levels, and pulse rate are the sensors connected to the person's body (body monitoring) [2], [3] [4]. Sensors placed throughout the patient's ambient location (environment monitoring) collect temperature data, lighting, moisture, Geo-location, body posture, motion, SPO2, atmospheric pressure, and CO2 [5].

The work given in [6] provides a mobility-aware architecture that incorporates ideas such as clouds, fog, and network virtualization, as well as an IoT level dubbed MobiIoST. The study investigated a situation in which a sensing layer made up of many sensor such as body temp, heartbeat, and cardiac output is used to monitor a patient's vital signs. Even while the patient is in the ambulance, such data may be captured and made accessible to medical personnel. The key concern is conveying this information on the go. Information connections frequently fail, compromising the availability and consistency of data. The findings established a framework for addressing this issue through the use of an IoT Layers, a Fog Layers, a Cloud Layers, as well as an Edge Layers.

In [7], the researchers suggest a fog-based framework for real-time job scheduling. The primary difficulty is that some healthcare information, such as an ECG signal, is time-sensitive. By employing fog cloud hosting, time limitations become even more difficult to meet. As a result, more healthcare awareness is necessary. For each key work including various types of knowledge such as pulse, electrocardiogram, and others. Job sequencing and task scheduling concerns are explored. To address a variety of scenarios, the authors employed many standard job scheduling methods, including the Earliest Priority is given to deadlines (EDF), shortest slack time (SSF), and shortest workload (SWF). All methods are applied to each case in order to choose the most appropriate one. Experiments were conducted with a fog-based cloud service, examining the storage and latency of data using publicly available datasets. Three distinct configurations of the Fog Node were used in each scenario, each with a distinct price. Evaluation of performance demonstrated that the suggested framework solution outperforms conventional approaches in terms of cost.

The articles [8] demonstrate also that SWITCH framework is effective in service observation via adapting instruments, growth target scheduling, and quality of service applications. Unfortunately, no one particular approach in health were selected as a standard.

Nowadays, modern technology has opened a new era of industrial growth. The use of novel technology [7 like the internet of things (IoT), data analytics, artificial intelligence (AI), and cloud computing has created a new form of industrial activities dubbed the Industry 4.0 (see Figure 5.2).

As per Yang et al. [9], the clinical wound has improved significantly as a result of emerging technology assistance from these growing sectors. This is referred to as Healthcare 4.0. It is described as a continuous (but innovative) transformation of the entire healthcare system, encompassing medical devices, hospital treatment,

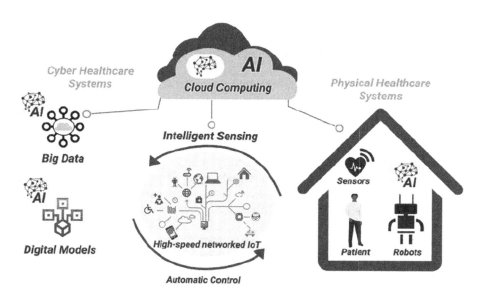

FIGURE 5.2 Integration of technology in a healthcare 4.0 context. This graphic has been taken from Ref. [9].

residential care, logistic, and a healthy lifestyle environment. This Healthcare 4.0 idea entails a paradigm shift in terms of sensors, data transformation, and data interpretation. It is mainly based on continuous measurement of a patient's health and system-to-system communication.

Hamdi [10] propose an Internet of Things-based, fog-based, and cloud-based home healthcare solution. The system's architecture facilitates local and distant monitoring using sensor networks and an Android App. This smartphone application serves as the Fog Nodes, monitoring the atmosphere within these nursing homes and collecting vital indicators through a sensor.

5.3 LAYOUT OF A HEALTHCARE SUPERVISORY SYSTEM

The design of IoT-enabled healthcare supervision system must be mobile and connect to nearby sensors through the internet. The supervisory systems' characteristics include mobility due to their small weight, a long battery life profile, a first aid crisis pushbutton, and a self-checking information user interface. Additionally, sensor and health care systems should function in an inconspicuous manner with respect to the current way of life. This system must ensure that both hardware and software components are genuine, secure, and diagnostically valid. Additionally, indigenous communication and ambient intelligence between healthcare processes and home-care supervision systems are necessary in clinical settings, as is a deep integration of wireless sensor technologies into another neighborhoods. These are the key aspects of IoT-based system applications in terms of laying the technological groundwork for ambient intelligence deployment.

The Internet of Things-based system is divided into basic three components: the patient's surroundings, cloud or fog healthcare facilities, and the hospitals. These components fulfil the functional needs of the solution and operate together to provide a monitoring system and effective care for people in serious condition.

The fundamental objective of the proposed Internet of Things-based healthcare system is to enable monitoring systems for patients who are in a life-threatening condition. This platform is built on the Internet of Things and connects patients, clinicians, and ambulance services in order to encourage improved treatment and rapid response to preventative and reactionary emergencies. Compatibility, safety, performance, and availability are all addressed. Remote Patient and Environmental Monitor, Patient Healthcare Data Processing, Patient Health Standardized Clinical, and Crisis and Strategic Planning are all needs for this platform [14].

Figure 5.3 illustrates a basic depiction of a remote monitoring system. Wearable sensors that collect physiologic and movement data, enabling for both the observation of a sufferer's status. Different sensors are installed depending on the medical application. Patient monitoring (e.g. cardiac output and breathing rate) would be also used to monitor the patient with heart problems or congestive heart failure who were undergoing therapeutic intervention. Sensors for recording movement data would be used in a variety of applications, including tracking the success of home-based rehabilitation therapies for stroke survivors and the usage of mobility assistance equipment by older persons. Wireless communication is used to provide patient data to a cell telephone or access point, which then relays it to a distant center through the Internet.

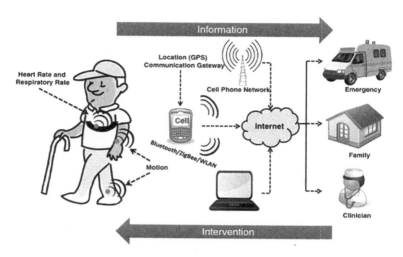

FIGURE 5.3   Design of a healthcare supervisory system [16].

Emergency circumstances (e.g. falls) are identified throughout the system via data processing, and an alert message is delivered to an urgent service department to give rapid help to patients. Relatives and caregivers are contacted in the event of an emergency, but may also be contacted in other circumstances, such as when the patient needs assistance taking his/her prescriptions. Clinical professionals can monitor a patient's state remotely and be notified if a clinic management has to be taken.

5.3.1   SENSOR DATA READING

Remote Patients and Surroundings Monitoring entails the collection of data via various sensors to the human body and even in the patient's environment (at home or in the intensive care unit). Clinical personnel (physicians and nurses) use the sensor data for health therapy and emergency alert reasons. Thus, the sensors linked to the person's body offer electrocardiogram, blood pressure and blood sugar, pulse rate, oxygen levels, temperature, respiratory rate, and capnography information (see Figure 5.4). The environmental sensors collect data on the temperature, location (latitude and longitude), and humidity of the surrounding area. This is critical because temperature and humidity management can have a direct effect on the patient's therapy. In terms of location, it aids in the ambulance service's speedy response. As a result, because the patient is at residence just not in a hospital, that is a more regulated setting, this ambience information is more crucial for optimal treatment and complements the remote monitoring given by this platform.

There are additional sensors that communicate wirelessly with embedded systems in situations when a wire connection is inconvenient, such as vibration sensors.

This innovation, illustrated in Figure 5.5, permits the capture of clinical data and its wireless transfer to a data acquisition system through a low-power radio. Microelectromechanical system (MEMS) manufacturing advancements are critical

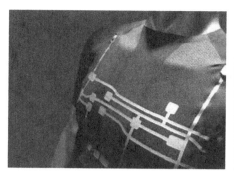
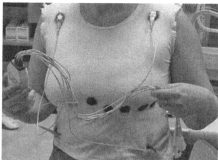

FIGURE 5.4   Sensing shirt wireless and wired.

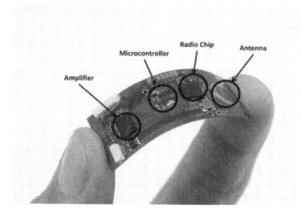

FIGURE 5.5   IMEC's flexible wireless ECG sensor has a fully working microprocessor [16].

for rehabilitation applications. MEMS enables the construction of extremely small inertial sensors for use in motor function and other health monitoring systems. Through the use of batch manufacturing techniques, the size and cost of sensors have been considerably decreased.

Traditionally used adhesive sensors for electric heart activity that are slathered on the skin have a limited lifespan owing to contact gel dehydration, skin shifting, and other factors. Nowadays, the tendency is to employ a new method of measuring that involves the use of a conducting polymer-based electrode that is covered by any form of flexible t-shirt. Polymer-based electrodes are used to measure ECGs or other bio signals with any number of leads, and they are wirelessly linked directly to a t-shirt pin terminal. That method is preferred because it provides long-term stability for electric signals conduction and scanning [15]. The integrated healthcare monitoring systems are capable of detecting falls and body postures. Numerous old adults struggle with balance and subsequent falls, which is dangerous on a vicariously unsafe level. The next issue is physics-based, and late-stage osteoporosis is highly harmful in contexts, not for survival, but for fatigue, hunger, pain, stress, and immobility if they truly live alone. They produce a deadly situation with a decreased chance of distress call when combined.

These sensors wouldn't need to be in close proximity to or constant contact with the human skin, as this creates pain again for person. If the user is calm and continues to wear the smart clothing for a lengthy period of time, untrustworthy connections formed through the user's motions will be enough to capture adequate data. As with conventional clothes, smart clothing may be customized for an individual.

5.3.2   DATA COMMUNICATIONS INFRASTRUCTURE

The next critical component of an environmental supervisory system is effective data transmission between sensors and the processing system. In the majority of medical applications, data transfer may be accomplished wirelessly, increasing viability and comfort in long-term user monitoring. In general, IoT communication protocols are categorized as follows: (1) The low-power wide area network (LPWAN) and (2) The short range network (SRN) protocols that provide adequate data transfer rates for continuous delivery of essential user important status information [5].

5.3.2.1   Low Power Wide Area Network (LPWAN)

SigFox: Indeed, SigFox is a low-power wireless standard for connecting the communication systems of a diverse range of low-power devices, including such sensor and machine-to-machine (M2M) applications. It is capable of transmitting small quantities of data across a distance of up to 50 kilometers. SigFox works throughout the Ultra Narrow Band (UNB) band of the electromagnetic spectrum. The technique is optimized for low-speed data transfers of up to 1000 bits per second and can be powered by a tiny battery [11].

Cellular: Cellular communication technology is a great replacement for applications that demand high data throughput and a power source for Internet of Things (IoT) applications that demand operation over greater distances. It may use GSM/3G/4G cellular connection capabilities to deliver stable high-speed internet connections. However, it consumes a lot of energy. As a consequence, it is incompatible with machine-to-machine or local area network connectivity [11].

5.3.2.2   Network with a Short Range

6LowPAN: 6LowPAN is a defined internetworking protocol based on IP; it is the first and most commonly used standard in the field of IoT communication protocols. It is capable of being directly connected to some other Internet protocol without the use of intermediary entities such as translations gateways or proxies. It offers 2128 IP addresses, which is more than enough.

Zig Bee: The Zig Bee protocol based on IEEE802.15.4, a low-power wireless networking standard. Zig Bee was created as a reference to produce increased, low-cost communication systems with the goal of building personal area networks (PANs) using small, low-power digitized radios capable of delivering data over long distances. Simultaneously, it will be employed in applications requiring a low data rate, increased battery performance, and secured networking devices.

BLE: BLE is commonly referred to it as Bluetooth smart, and it is a crucial standard in Internet of Things (IoT) applications. It is optimized for short-range, low-bandwidth, and low-latency Internet of Things applications. The benefits of BLE over conventional Bluetooth are that it consumes less power.

RFID: RFID consists of two components: a reader and a small radio frequency transponder referred to as an RF tag. This tag is digitally embedded using unique data that permits remote reading. RFID tag systems are classified into two types: active reading tagging system and passive reading tag systems. Active tags require batteries, are more expensive, and function at longer wavelengths, whereas passive tags work at shorter wavelengths and do not require a power source. Because RFID data is static and must be programmed into to the tags, it cannot be used instantly for measuring or diagnostic purposes. RFID is used in a wide variety of Internet of Things (IoT) applications, such as digital commerce, healthcare, homeland security, and agriculture.

NFC: NFC is a near-field communication (NFC) technology that enables data transfer among devices simply by touching or placing devices within a few inches of each other. NFC is a near-field communication (NFC) technology that is analogous to RFID. Additionally to identification, it is utilized for more sophisticated two-way communication. The NFC tag stores a finite amount of data. This tag can also be read-only (which RFID tags are designed to be) or it can be rewritable and replaced back by the device.

Z-Wave: Z-Wave is a limited MAC protocol that connects 30–50 nodes via wireless automation. It has been used to communicate with the Internet of Things (IoT), most notably in the intelligent home or small business sectors. This method is optimized for brief data streams for point-to-point communication within a 30 meter radius at a relatively modest transmit power of up to 100 kbps.

Previous research on existing wireless communication protocols has concentrated on the most prevalent technologies, including Bluetooth Low Energy (BLE), Wi-Fi with IEEE 802.11 standard, WPAN (Zig Bee/IEEE 802.15.4), and WiMAX (IEEE 802.15.4). (Near Field Communication).

Figure 5.6 shows the different wireless technologies available for use and the choice of wireless data transmission technology is determined by the amount of data and the distance of transmission between sensors and IoT systems. Communication tests were performed to validate the usability of home-care software. We applied the BLE to monitor key parameters. Additionally, we evaluated Zig Bee technology and data transmission over a medium distance range, with disappointing results.

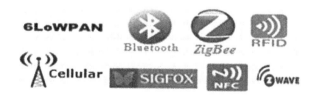

FIGURE 5.6 Wireless communication technology.

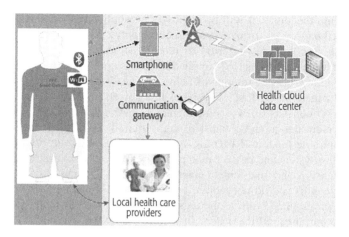

FIGURE 5.7   Sensors' data communication with the cloud [13].

5.3.3 COMMUNICATION WITH CLOUD SERVICES

Healthcare big data may be kept for an extended length of time with the assistance of a cloud service, and cloud-based big data analytics may significantly boost the intellectual and communication power of a humanoid robotics.

When a person goes outdoors (as shown in Figure 5.7), his or her smartphone acts as a personal gateway, transmitting sensory cardiac information to the server via Bluetooth. The smartphone, as the primary communication link between wearable devices and the clouds, also saves and analyses health information locally. Additionally, medical monitoring applications help consumers to have a better understanding of their health status. Certain users, such as the aged, children, handicapped, and individuals with Alzheimer's disease, use smartphones rarely or have issues. Network nodes must be put in areas where such users engage in routine activities. As a result, low-power Wi-Fi is the optimal solution for connecting smart garments to the cloud in this scenario. Or we can use both combinations, Wi-Fi as well mobile gateway for data communication with cloud system [17].

Finally, when data is gathered from multiple sources, it is stored and analysed via a cloud service. Following data processing, analytical results are communicated to multiple components from the inside of the healthcare data center, including medical advisors, emergency medical assistance, robots, and family members.

All sensors linked to the human body act as a protracted data source, which is essential for gathering large amounts of health data. To provide a positive user experience, the suggested system might incorporate healthcare robotics. A robotic arm with a humanoid shell, for example, could deliver more friendly and tailored healthcare services. For instance, if a user has a heart attack and lost linguistic capabilities, a healthcare robotic can transmit video and images to a faraway medical facility or close family members. Additionally, whenever emotion-aware services are needed, a robot capable of walking is critical for emotional connection. Thus, integrating smart clothes with a humanoid robot benefits the system's interoperability in a variety of complex settings.

5.3.4 ROLE OF SOFTWARE

Each system is only as good as the software that runs on it. Additionally, the software capability enhances the power of IoT systems. Again from start, software controls sensor sensing via regularity of input, filtration, and packet data creation. The subsequent process is data transmission between the transceiver and the quantity of data transported, followed by packets control to store the data and assure its dependability and security. IoT systems collect data and collect information for the purpose of making an input sequence, setting or assigning them to a healthcare expert such as a medical supervisor or administering help first. Overall strength of a software component is proportional to the size of the system's infrastructure. The implementation of that aspect of measurement is far more involved than the implementation of the equipment.

5.3.5 SUPERVISORY HEALTH SYSTEM

All monitoring systems, but especially healthcare supervisory systems, have the objective of communicating urgent situations and safeguarding first-aid treatment. Integration of hardware and software that interact with the software agents at each level is necessary for the purpose of processing the adaptive remote diagnostic system. Data measuring is a challenge of accurate sharing information in the home healthcare application. An ECG signal across 12 lead measurement provides a wealth of useful information about the patient's health status. It is responsible for around 82 percent of all health issues. As a result, ECG analysis is a critical component of the signal interpretation. We evaluated signals recorded by an IoT system using new mathematical methodologies including practical expert system decision trees.

Patient monitoring systems are gaining traction as a means of diagnosing and treating patients, while also lowering inpatient expenditures. Telehealth solutions enable the integration of many clinical goals: preventive, diagnostic, treatment, admittance, and care homes. Since people actively participate around their own therapy, the out-of-clinic method fosters a stronger clinician connection. In this manner, not only can the patient's health status be monitored, but also the effectiveness of care may be evaluated, with the goal of eventually modifying pharmacological therapies.

Severe and life-threatening events are communicated via call or text to a supervisory center, emergency medical aid, medial advisor and others such as family members or neighbours. Concurrently, there must be the ability to communicate measured data from the user to the supervisory center through LAN, Wi-Fi, or 5G connection (see Figure 5.8).

A supervisory core in collaboration with local health care providers is able to identify risk factors that individuals may encounter when visiting a local health provider. Using this IoT-based system, the supervisory central communicates with the health datacenter via Bluetooth or Wi-Fi modules. These modules communicate with the health datacenter via a communication gateway or a smartphone.

This user-provided representative data set provides clinical information about the true plunge risk, which is used to calibrate the sensing settings in the event of a false alarm. After receiving a demand from a medical sight at the supervisory center, it is

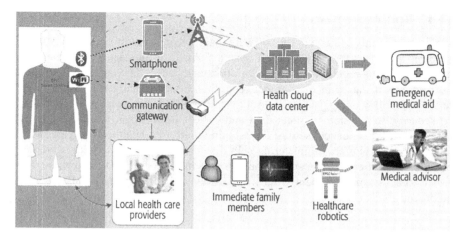

FIGURE 5.8   General configuration of remote diagnosis [13].

required to alter data in the decisions program in the IoT device at the user level via a variety of techniques, including cellular GSM.

The diagnostic information is saved on the centralized terminal server. The central terminal system is equipped with software programs that perform various diagnostic tests on the embedded computer. It is impossible to measure direct parameters in home care applications. There are only measurable indirect parameters that provide us with knowledge about the problem that is not included in the measured data. A treatment such as shocks or feedback to the user may be used to break the situation. As an illustration, sleep apnea is unquestionably harmful in half-slim old individuals.

The hospital in which such IoT-based healthcare was implemented is now treating patients infected with the Corona Infectious Diseases (COVID-19) outbreak. Given the nature of the disease, it is important to maintain a low level of contact with affected individuals, since physical contact with people infected poses hazards to the health care team [18], and thus, telemedicine has emerged as a significant ally in the battle against the illness. When ICU clinical team members utilize the system, they are not required to have physical communication with the patient to monitor vital signs, which lowers the risk of infection, particularly among healthcare personnel who are on the frontlines of disease prevention.

5.4   CONCLUSION

In recent years, healthcare systems around the world have undergone significant changes. A smart healthcare system powered by the Internet of Things has added a new dimension to drugs and treatment in hospitals. This study focuses on the right medicine for a patient. This study will aid older adults who require regular medication monitoring. This project incorporates a cloud service for storing and analyzing data and interpreting information, a mail transmission protocol, a temperature sensor, an

ECG sensor, a blood pressure sensor, and a heart pulse sensor for proper monitoring of the patient's body.

REFERENCES

[1] Gulraiz J. Joyia, Rao M. Liaqat, Aftab Farooq, and Saad Rehman, Internet of Medical Things (IoMT): Applications, Benefits and Future Challenges in Healthcare Domain, Journal of Communications Vol. 12, No. 4, April 2017.

[2] G. Yang, L. Xie, M. Mantysalo, X. Zhou, Z. Pang, L. D. Xu, S. Kao-Walter, Q. Chen, and L.-R. Zheng, "A health-IoT platform based on the integration of intelligent packaging, unobtrusive bio-sensor, and intelligent medicine box," *IEEE Trans. Ind. Informat.*, vol. 10, no. 4, pp. 2180–2191,Nov. 2014.

[3] A. J. Jara, M. A. Zamora-Izquierdo, and A. F. Skarmeta, "Interconnection framework for mHealth and remote monitoring based on the Internet of Things," *IEEE J. Sel. Areas Commun.*, vol. 31, no. 9, pp. 47–65, Sep. 2013.

[4] J. H. Abawajy and M. M. Hassan, "Federated Internet of Things and cloud computing pervasive patient health monitoring system," *IEEE Commun. Mag.*, vol. 55, no. 1, pp. 48–53, Jan. 2017.

[5] M. Chen, Y. Ma, Y. Li, D. Wu, Y. Zhang, and C.-H. Youn, "Wearable 2.0: Enabling human-cloud integration in next generation healthcare systems," *IEEE Commun. Mag.*, vol. 55, no. 1, pp. 54–61, Jan. 2017.

[6] S. Ghosh, A. Mukherjee, S. K. Ghosh, and R. Buyya, "Mobi-IoST: Mobility-aware cloud-fog-edge-IoT collaborative framework for timecritical applications," *IEEE Trans. Netw. Sci. Eng.*, vol. 7, no. 4, pp. 2271–2285, Oct. 2020.

[7] Q.-U.-A. Mastoi, T. Ying Wah, R. Gopal Raj, and A. Lakhan, "A novel cost-efficient framework for critical heartbeat task scheduling using the Internet of medical things in a fog cloud system," *Sensors*, vol. 20, no. 2, p. 441, Jan. 2020.

[8] P. Tefanic, M. Cigale, A. C. Jones, L. Knight, I. Taylor, C. Istrate, G. Suciu, A. Ulisses, V. Stankovski, S. Taherizadeh, G. F. Salado, S. Koulouzis, P. Martin, and Z. Zhao, "SWITCH workbench: A novel approach for the development and deployment of time-critical microservice-based cloudnative applications," *Future Gener. Comput. Syst.*, vol. 99, pp. 197–212, Oct. 2019.

[9] G. Yang, Z. Pang, M. J. Deen, M. Dong, Y.-T. Zhang, N. Lovell, and A. M. Rahmani, "Homecare robotic systems for healthcare 4.0: Visions and enabling technologies," *IEEE J. Biomed. Health Informat.*, vol. 24, no. 9, pp. 2535–2549, Sep. 2020.

[10] H. Ben Hassen, N. Ayari, and B. Hamdi, "A home hospitalization system based on the Internet of Things, fog computing and cloud computing," *Informat. Med. Unlocked*, vol. 20, Jan. 2020, Art. no. 100368.

[11] Samie, F., Bauer, L. & Henkel, J. 2016. IoT technologies for embedded computing: A survey. Hardware/Software Codesign and System Synthesis (CODES+ ISSS), 2016 International Conference on: 1–10

[12] Ghamari, M., Janko, B., Sherratt, R.S., Harwin, W., Piechockic, R. and Soltanpur, C., 2016. A survey on wireless body area networks for ehealthcare systems in residential environments. *Sensors*, 16(6), p. 831.

[13] Chen, M., Ma, Y., Li, Y., Wu, D., Zhang, Y. and Youn, C.H., 2017. Wearable 2.0: Enabling human-cloud integration in next generation healthcare systems. *IEEE Communications Magazine*, 55(1), pp. 54–61

[14] M. S. Hossain and G. Muhammad, "Cloud-Assisted Industrial Internet of Things (IIoT)-Enabled Framework for Health Monitoring", *Computer Networks*, vol. 101, pp. 192–202, 2016.

[15]　S.-H. Seo, J.-W. Jang and S.-W. Jang, "Design and Implementation of a Smart Clothing System Coping with Emergency Status", *Int'l. Info. Inst. Tokyo*, vol. 19, no. 1, pp. 175, 2016.

[16]　Patel, S., Park, H., Bonato, P., Chan, L. and Rodgers, M., 2012. A review of wearable sensors and systems with application in rehabilitation. *Journal of neuroengineering and rehabilitation*, 9(1), pp. 1–17.

[17]　Gupta, P., Shukla, M., Arya, N., Singh, U. and Mishra, K., 2022. Let the Blind See: An AIIoT-Based Device for Real-Time Object Recognition with the Voice Conversion. In *Machine Learning for Critical Internet of Medical Things* (pp. 177–198). Springer, Cham.

[18]　Gupta, P., Sharma, V. and Varma, S., 2021. People detection and counting using YOLOv3 and SSD models. *Materials Today: Proceedings*.

6 Energy Harvesting for IoT Networks in Smart and Intelligent Networks

Yogita Thareja, Kamal Kumar Sharma, and Parulpreet Singh
Lovely Professional University, Phagwara, India

CONTENTS

6.1   INTRODUCTION

The Internet of things (IoT), also thought of as the Web of things, is the coordinated interconnection of traditional things. In IoT, things are the contraptions (physical or virtual) that are somewhat related through the web, like 4G connected with telephones. These contraptions have a remarkable ID that recollects them unexpectedly shockingly. It isn't restricted to contraptions or devices; it also allows gadgets to communicate (obviously or by implication) with one another by sending/getting information. Contraptions ought to be able to eliminate data by sifting, dealing with and gathering information, and after information has been obtained from that data the gadgets play out their various activities. Some properties of the IoT frameworks are Dynamic nature, Self-evolving, Self-putting together, and so on. For the most part, IoT contraptions are energized by batteries. A significant limit of gadgets fueled by a battery is limited to battery life since when IoT gadgets speak with one another, a lot of energy is used and so the gadgets work for a restricted length of time – just as long as the battery endures. The arrangement for this issue is to utilize replaceable batteries. This arrangement of trading batteries might be successful for little IoT frameworks; however, for huge IoT frameworks, this arrangement isn't successful due to the expense of keeping up with and supplanting billions of batteries being extremely high. A promising answer to this issue is energy harvesting. IoT is a savvy

DOI: 10.1201/9781003145035-6

network foundation wherein an enormous number of interestingly recognizable things or items (e.g. remote gadgets) are interconnected to perform complex errands in helpful habits [1]–[4]. As of late, IoT applications dependent on heterogeneous remote sensor organization wireless sensor network (WSN) design are drawing in huge consideration from the examination of the local area. By empowering simple access and cooperation with articles, the WSN-based (IoT) worldview is tracking down practices in numerous spaces, like Keen Home, Brilliant Medical care, Keen Transportation, Savvy City, and Shrewd Framework [4]. The harvesting of energy is the most common way of extracting energy from at least one natural (sun-based, wind, radiofrequency, and so on) or other energy sources (body heat, finger strokes, foot strikes, and so forth), collecting them and changing them into usable electrical energy. This harvested electrical energy controls the IoT gadgets and increases the lifetime of the IoT framework. The harvester architectures of energy are (i) Harvest and Use: without a moment to spare, energy is gathered and straightaway utilized, (ii) Harvest-Store-Use at whatever point accessible, energy is gathered and stored, which can then be utilized in the future at the appropriate time. In Harvest and Use architecture, the collected energy is used straightaway to drive the framework. Whenever harvested energy isn't sufficient, the framework will stay out of gear state. In Harvest-Store-Use architecture, the gathered energy can straightaway power the framework and, when the accessibility of harvested energy is greater than the current need of the framework, then, at that point, the remaining energy is stored for some time in the future. On the other hand, energy can likewise be stored until adequate energy has been stored for framework activity. The energy is put away in optional capacity, which is utilized when essential stockpiling (battery) is depleted [5]. The rise of cutting edge EH procedures has advanced an outlook change in the plan of steering conventions for the remote network including harvesting of energy from "aware energy" to "energy-collecting mindful" [6]– [12]. The ordinarily utilized methodology in the greater part of these steering calculations is given in terms of the algorithm of a minimum path named Dijkstra's shortest path algorithm to track down the base course to advance information parcels from the originator to the endpoints [13]. The energy harvesting sources are utilized to expand the lifetime and effectiveness of the IoT framework. The energy sources utilized for energy harvesting components are, all things considered, natural sources like sun-powered, wind and so forth, or other energy sources like temperature contrast, movement, footfall, breathing, and mobile devices [14–17].

6.2   LITERATURE SURVEY

Concerning "energy – reaping mindful" coordinating strategies, the author in [18] presents the Energy-Opportunistic Weighted Minimum Energy calculation that works out the expense of all tactile harvests utilizing reasonable power and energy assortment rate. Activity [19] promotes an algorithm to route data randomly in a minimum path recovery time. In this case, cost metrics are seen as part of the energy used to harness the package (referred to as package power) and energy harvesting rate. The hub gets short lessons in the sink related to the marked cost metric. A package from the hub will be sent for its intended purpose using the visible cost link base. In [20], the choice of direction depends on the expense metaphor which includes the energy consumed and the accumulated energy wasted as a result of cheating. In [21], the smart energy harvesting routing (SEHR) protocol is in high demand. The proposed power harvesting steering assembly in [22] is in line with the environmental control approach. This conference uses a game guessing method to consider both the strength and harvesting power of all nodes to improve the network environment. By checking the speed of energy consumed and gathered by every one of the harbours at various times, the transmission force of the node is constrained by helping it power frameworks and its neighbours. Even though the previously mentioned controlling insights can decrease power utilization and expand the life expectancy of nodes, they actually have their inner issues. Concerning the idea of energy assortment, [18] and [20] won't consider the genuine measure of energy gathered during the reap. It is designed [23] to use stable charging standards for all hubs in the organization. In addition, due to the lack of collected power tests, most current regulatory agreements are unable to adjust or manage stochastic attributes for continuous sources. One additional limitation is the organization of the power source setting alone for power collection. It is noteworthy that non-biological energy sources are subject to climate, seasons, and permanent cycles, in addition, to even higher / no higher periods. At present, a single power source system may not be sufficient to extend the life of the node, especially in the evening (i.e. solar-powered EH) or at idle times (i.e. EH-based vehicle). Therefore, another partial system that combines a few different types of power collectors with a certified node should be considered as the growth rate of new energy harvesting directors [24].

From a regulatory perspective, the control tables used to develop masses in the aforementioned directional figures are based on global network status data. In different climates, however, global data may not be able to adapt to types of energy sensor hubs (e.g. lingering, devoured, and collected energy levels). Therefore, it is important to create control tables using location data, especially with the distributed style of applications (IoT).

It is required to set another target for harnessing the power of various IoT organizations. The proposed accounting centers focus on EE issues, QoS, and lifelong enhancements under the conditions of IoT applications and stochastic power collection processes. Directing options further consider the effects of both types of one type, half-breed design.

6.3   PROPOSED MODEL

In this model, the sensor nodes can be categorized as primary and secondary users. Sensor nodes that generate information parcels will be sent to the sink, while secondary users assist key hubs in sending parcels to the sink by combining multiple jumps. As an entry into the IoT framework, the sink removes data from information collected from the sensory hub and further transfers it to the server farm.

We process the WSN jump often consisting of a few sensory radio notes that include both primary and secondary users and a sink which is displayed in Figure 6.1. A keen city system is taken where the CR nodes are dispersed over a wide area randomly. Unlimited power is given to the sink. Cognitive radio nodes may collect energy from the sun, vibrations of the mobile vehicle, or from any other source.

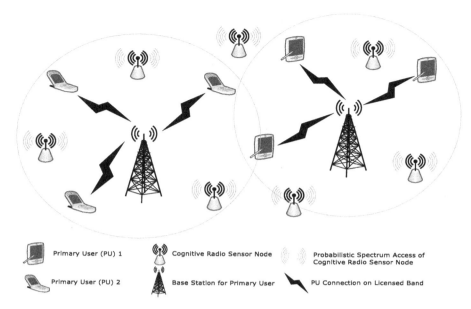

FIGURE 6.1 Network model.

Figure 6.1 depicts the network model. The framework model can be displayed as a chart with a graph G having N number of nodes and E number of edges and can be designated as G(v, e) where:

v- number of CR nodes and sink
e- link between CR nodes

The cognitive sensor nodes are fueled by sustainable power sources as displayed in Figure 6.2 and Figure 6.3 respectively. The CR node structure comprises a miniature regulator (low-power) termed a micro-controller, a low-power RF handset (an IEEE 802.15.4-based) [24], an energy stockpiling gadget (a powered battery), and an energy harvester. To productively use the approaching energy, the "harvest – store-use" convention allows the CR node to store energy initially and then utilize the energy which was harvested.

We included the accompanying designs for every one of these EH strategies:

1. Energy harvesting technique using Sun's energy: Here energy is harvested by using the sun's energy. The size of a solar panel for harvesting energy from sunlight is 50mm×50mm. Figure 6.2 depicts the solar-based energy harvesting.

2. Energy harvested technique for mobile vehicle: On a fundamental level, each moving vehicle out and about provides its tyre's vibration and weight onto an energy gatherer set on the blacktop to deliver a proportion of force shown in Figure 6.3. The energy associated with the hub's battery by a connection

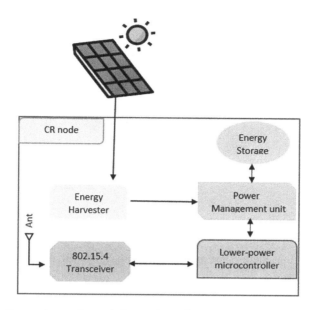

FIGURE 6.2   Energy harvesting technique using solar energy.

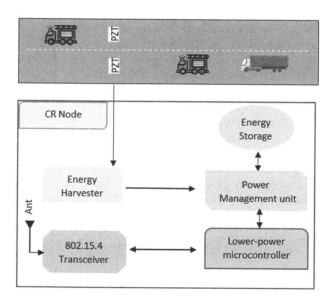

FIGURE 6.3   Energy harvested technique for a vehicle.

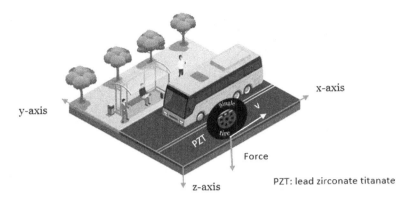

FIGURE 6.4 Roadside energy harvesting mechanism.

link and the energy loss presented by the physical link is expected to be unimportant.

In this chapter, we foster a successful enhancement of the harvesting algorithm based on an energy-aware routing algorithm, alluded to as EHRA (energy harvesting routing algorithm) (see Figure 6.4). Utilizing the EH methods, our calculation resolves the issues of energy consumption and packet loss ratio, which increases the lifetime expansion and the heterogeneity of IoT gadgets. Specifically, the algorithm here chooses the most effective courses by utilizing two distinct cost measurements characterised as mixes of the harvested and the leftover energy at hubs. The commitments of this paper are summed up as follows:

- We, while also considering the issues of energy harvesting and packet loss ratio for IoT applications, foster the enhancement of an energy-harvesting-aware routing algorithm working at the organization layer. The proposed algorithm can proficiently adjust to the shifting traffic load produced when applicable to cognitive radio sensor nodes.
- We propose another energy expectation model for the appearance of harvested energy at the hubs. The stochastic attributes of the surrounding energy sources are considered in the model.

In this work, we think about the accompanying three situations.

Scheme 1: Each cognitive radio node is all the while outfitted with two kinds of the harvester to gain energy from the sun and mobile vehicles.
Scheme 2: The cognitive radio nodes are similarly isolated into three gatherings of one, and two, which utilize the energy harvesting using the sun's energy and energy harvesting using mobile vehicles individually.
Scheme 3: A single source CR node may harvest energy in three modes, either utilizing the energy from the sun, from the mobile vehicle, or any other source.

6.3.1   Energy Consumption Model

To plan the proposed energy consumption model, it is important to decide the energy devoured by every hub to handle the packet.

The nodes need the energy to send, get, or advance parcels in the chosen way. Furthermore, the node needs to use energy to tune in for an appearance bundle or hang tight for an approaching occasion.

For processing a packet the energy consumption may be written as:

$$E_c^1 = E_l^1 + E_{tx}^1 + E_{rx}^1 + E_{rl}^1 \qquad (1)$$

E_c^1 = Energy collecting of CR node 1
$E_l^1, E_{tx}^1, E_{rx}^1, E_{rl}^1$ = Energy consumption for listening, transmitting, receiving, and resting.

Energy harvesting cognitive radio networks include many approaches like Kalman filtering (which is stochastic) and time series forecasting, etc. Here the mixture of both is taken where Kalman filtering is taken for the arrival energy from different surrounding sources and time series forecasting is used for mobile nodes.

$$x_k = Ax_{k-1} + Bu_k + w_k \qquad (2)$$

$$z_k = Hx_k + v_k \qquad (3)$$

A, B, H – Transition matrix
u_k – Input vector (control)
x_k, z_k – True state of the system

Here we are using the super enhancement of harvesting algorithm based on energy-aware, which is the enhancement of energy harvesting aware routing algorithm. It includes two selections: path selection and forwarder selection.

In the path selection phase, a minimum distance is selected for the nodes with i, j and k vectors as explained:

$$C_{min} = \min\left(C_{i,j}, C_{i,k}\right) \forall i, j, k \in V \qquad (4)$$

C_{min} – minimum distance

In forwarder selection, the CR node selects its minimum distance node and forwards the message to the next nearest node which is in its range.

6.3.2   Measures of Energy Harvesting

Introducing the ranges of battery for a CR node, the battery for the CR node may be divided into three locales as displayed in Figure 6.5. Level three is the base strength degree to assure that the CR hub works properly with four running modes (i.e. getting, sending, inactive tuning in, and resting). The remaining energy of a battery is shown in Figure 6.5. We examine three parts:

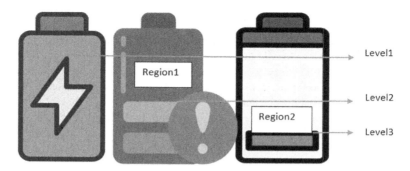

FIGURE 6.5   Remaining energy of battery.

Here L1 L2 and L3 are regarded as Level 1, Level 2, and Level 3 respectively:

- Part 1: L 2 < Ei ≤ L1
  The remaining energy is adequately high for the hubs to keep up with their typical tasks. Henceforth, the energy collecting process isn't needed in the present situation.
- Part 2: L3 < Ei ≤ L2
  For this situation, we exploit the resting time frame to empower hubs so that they could harvest more energy. With this, the hubs not just decrease the utilization of energy, but in addition gather a limited quantity of energy from encompassing energy sources. Thus, they can broaden their lifetime.
- Part 3: 0 < Ei ≤ L3
  In this situation, there may not be sufficient energy for the hubs to keep up with their ordinary tasks. Subsequently, the hub should briefly put off its handsets and come in the state of resting mode to save energy.

6.4   RESULTS AND DISCUSSION

This unit gives a thorough experimental study using the proposed enhancement energy harvesting aware routing algorithm. The recommended model has been implemented in the MATLAB tool. Table 6.1 shows the simulation parameters used for the experimentation.

We have taken three cases here which are energy harvesting technique using Sun's energy, the energy harvested technique for mobile vehicles, and any other way. Let us consider any other way will be energy harvesting by using RF energy sources the BS which is deployed at the origin and a total number of nodes = {100, 200, 300, 400, 500} hubs haphazardly dispersed over a square district, each at first outfitted with 0.5 J of energy and has an information transmission pace of 2000 pieces for every bundle.

Each CH hub is served by an extraordinary EH hub, for the scope of EH rates somewhere in the range of 0.03W and 0.09W, in strides of 0. 02W (see Figure 6.6).

For this simulation, we have varied the EH rate for 500 sensor nodes. The first scenario (see Figure 6.7) considers the network without any harvesting node and the

TABLE 6.1
Simulation Parameters

Strategies	Parameter	Value
Apps- IoT	Packet size (*bits*)	1000
Apps- IoT	Traffic (packet / *s*)	[0.1:1.5]
Solar -based EH	Size of solar panel	50mm×50mm
EH technique for mobile vehicle	Weight (kg)	[1,890–2,100]
	Speed (m/s)	[5–25]
	Arrival time of vehicle(s)	[0.8–1.0]
Battery	Initial energy	1.2J
CR node	Voltage	3V
CR node	Number	100

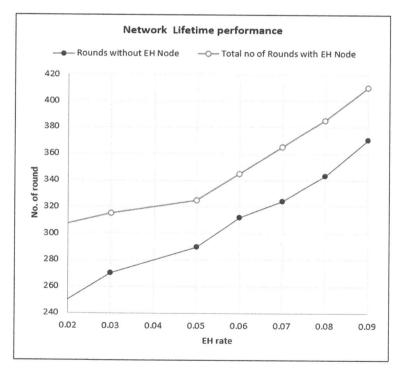

FIGURE 6.6 Energy consumption performance.

second scenario (see Figure 6.8) considers the sensor node with an energy harvesting node. The average network lifetime is obtained as 311 and 348 rounds for mentioned scenarios.

In this experiment, we measure the number of iterations taken to report the first dead node with and without the EH node for a varied number of nodes.

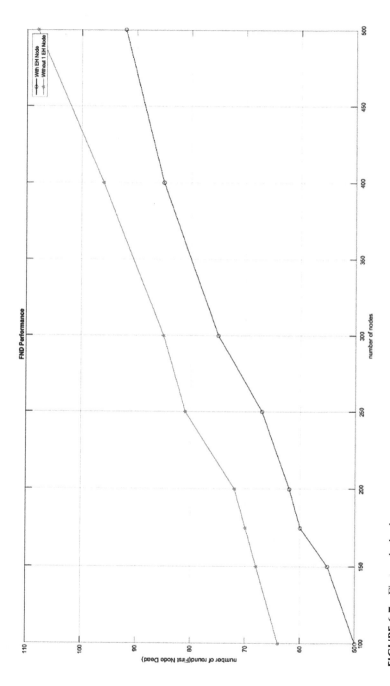

FIGURE 6.7 First node dead.

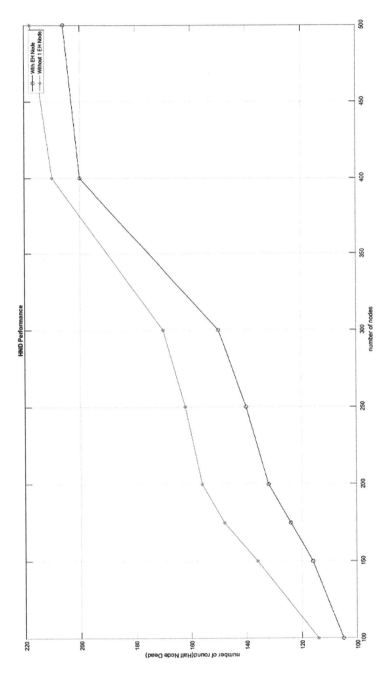

FIGURE 6.8 Half node dead scenario.

In this experiment, we measure the number of iterations taken to report the half number of a dead node with and without an EH node for a varied number of nodes.

The EH scenario achieves better performance. However, the clustering or multipath routing mechanisms can be incorporated to further evaluate the performance.

6.5 CONCLUSION

In this chapter, we have explored the issues of energy utilization and parcel loss proportion in a manner for IoT networks with two energy gathering methodologies: energy harvesting utilizing Sun's energy and energy harvesting utilizing the mobile vehicle. We propose an improvement of EHRA, to determine the issues of nature of administration. Results have been performed on MATLAB, which shows that the proposed is better when contrasted with the current plan. The results moreover show that the delivery of the hybrid plan with various energy sources is a capable, suitable and down-to-earth reply for QoS issues and similarly to expand the lifetime of devices in IoT associations.

REFERENCES

1. Kansal, A., Hsu, J., Zahedi, S., & Srivastava, M. B. (2007). "Power management in energy harvesting sensor networks. ACM Transactions on Embedded Computing Systems (TECS)", 6(4), 32.
2. A. Zanella, N. Bui, A. Castellani, L. Vangelista, and M. Zorzi, "Internet of Things for smart cities," vol. 1, no. 1, pp. 22–32, Feb 2014.
3. L. Atzori, A. Iera, and G. Morabito, "The Internet of Things: A survey," Computer Networks, vol. 54, no. 15, pp. 2787–2805, 2010.
4. P. Kamalinejad, C. Mahapatra, Z. Sheng, S. Mirabbasi, V. Leung, and Y. L. Guan, "Wireless energy harvesting for the Internet of Things," IEEE Commun. Mag., vol. 53, no. 6, pp. 102–108, Jun 2015.
5. Jiang, X., Polastre, J., & Culler, D. (2005, April). "Perpetual environmentally powered sensor networks. In Proceedings of the 4th international symposium on Information processing in sensor networks (p. 65). IEEE Press.
6. Z. Lu and Y. Wen, "Distributed algorithm for tree-structured data aggregation service placement in smart grid," IEEE Syst. J., vol. 8, no. 2, pp. 553–561, Jun 2014.
7. A. E. Zonouz, L. Xing, V. M. Vokkarane, and Y. Sun, "Hybrid wireless sensor networks: a reliability, cost, and energy-aware approach," IET Wireless Sensor Systems, vol. 6, no. 2, pp. 42–48, Jan 2016.
8. H. Chen, Y. Li, J. Rebelatto, B. Uchoa Filho, and B. Vucetic, "Harvest then cooperate: Wireless-powered cooperative communications," IEEE Trans. Signal Process., vol. 63, no. 7, pp. 1700–1711, Apr 2015.
9. R. Fedrizzi, K. Gomez, S. Kandeepan, T. Rasheed, and C. V. Saradhi, "Energy-aware routing in heterogeneous multi-hop public safety wireless networks," in Proc. of IEEE International Conference on Communications Workshops (ICC) 2014, Jun 2014, pp. 218–224.
10. A. Ahmed, K. A. Bakar, M. I. Channa, K. Haseeb, and A. W. Khan, "TERP: A trust and energy-aware routing protocol for wireless sensor network," IEEE Sensors J., vol. 15, no. 12, pp. 6962–6972, Dec 2015

11. Q. Tan, W. An, Y. Han, Y. Liu, S. Ci, F.-M. Shao, and H. Tang, "Energy harvesting aware topology control with power adaptation in wireless sensor networks," Ad Hoc Networks, vol. 27, pp. 44–56, 2015.

12. T. He, K. W. Chin, and S. Soh, "On wireless power transfer and max flow in rechargeable wireless sensor networks," vol. 4, pp. 4155–4167, Aug 2016.

13. F. Ye, A. Chen, S. Lu, and L. Zhang, "A scalable solution to minimum cost forwarding in large sensor networks," in Proc. of 10th Int'l. Conf. Comp. Commun. and Networks 2001, 2001, pp. 304–309.

14. Atallah, R., Khabbaz, M., & Assi, C. (2016). Energy harvesting in vehicular networks: a contemporary survey. IEEE Wireless Communications, 23(2), 70–77.

15. Cetinkaya, O., & Akan, O. B. (2017)." Electric-Field Energy Harvesting in Wireless Networks. IEEE Wireless Communications", 24(2), 34–41.

16. Sudevalayam, S., & Kulkarni, P. (2011)." Energy harvesting sensor nodes: Survey and implications. IEEE Communications Surveys & Tutorials", 13(3), 443–461.

17. Kulah, H., & Najafi, K. (2008)." Energy scavenging from low-frequency vibrations by using frequency up-conversion for wireless sensor applications". IEEE Sensors Journal, 8(3), 261–268.

18. L. Lin, N. B. Shroff, and R. Srikant, "Asymptotically optimal energy aware routing for multihop wireless networks with renewable energy sources," IEEE/ACM Trans. Netw., vol. 15, no. 5, pp. 1021–1034, Oct 2007

19. E. Lattanzi, E. Regini, A. Acquaviva, and A. Bogliolo, "Energetic sustainability of routing algorithms for energy-harvesting wireless sensor networks," Computer Communications, vol. 30, no. 14, pp. 2976–2986, 2007.

20. G. Martinez, S. Li, and C. Zhou, "Wastage-aware routing in energy harvesting Wireless Sensor Networks," IEEE Sensors J., vol. 14, no. 9, pp. 2967–2974, Sep 2014.

21. J. Bai, M. Fan, J. Yang, Y. Sun, and C. Phillips, "Smart energy harvesting routing protocol for WSN based E-health systems," in Proc. of the 2015 Workshop on Pervasive Wireless Healthcare (MobileHealth '15), 2015, pp. 23–28.

22. Q. Tan, W. An, Y. Han, Y. Liu, S. Ci, F.-M. Shao, and H. Tang, "Energy harvesting aware topology control with power adaptation in wireless sensor networks," Ad Hoc Networks, vol. 27, pp. 44–56, 2015.

23. T. He, K. W. Chin, and S. Soh, "On wireless power transfer and max flow in rechargeable wireless sensor networks," vol. 4, pp. 4155–4167, Aug 2016.

24. T. D. Nguyen, J. Y. Khan, and D. T. Ngo, "An effective energy harvesting-aware routing algorithm for WSN-based IoT applications," in Proc. of IEEE International Conference on Communications (ICC) 2017, May 2017, pp. 1–6.

25. Nguyen, T. D., Khan, J. Y., & Ngo, D. T. (2018). "A distributed energy-harvesting-aware routing algorithm for heterogeneous IoT networks". IEEE Transactions on Green Communications and Networking, 2(4), 1115–1127.

7 IoT Healthcare Applications

Shifa Manihar[1] and Tasneem Bano Rehman[2]
[1] Rajiv Gandhi Technical University, Bhopal, Madhya Pradesh, India
[2] Sage University, Bhopal, Madhya Pradesh, India

CONTENTS

DOI: 10.1201/9781003145035-7

7.1 INTRODUCTION

In the face of technology developments, appropriate medical facilities and resources are still not accessible to a large percentage of the population, especially those with low income and living in the countryside or remote areas. There is a crucial prerequisite for expansion of a low cost and highly reliable technology for monitoring healthcare for those with unbalanced regulatory body system, vulnerable to heart attacks or who may have suffered one before, critical body organ circumstances, chancy life-threatening disorder and athletes during training so as to recognize which training regimes will yield improved outcomes. The conventional healthcare monitoring systems consist of clinics, hospitals with big medical machinery comprising complex circuitry with high cost and power intake. The IoT-based healthcare system enables improved diagnostic equipment to provide enhanced therapy to patients and keen healthcare gadgets that give crucial indicators in real-time to enhance healthcare efficiency. Altogether IoT has many applications in healthcare for easing the work with and few listed below:

- Increase in overall reachability of healthcare service to all the sections of the society.
- Patients with critical health issue can be provided with continuous monitoring by the medical staff.
- Reducing the delay in the transmission of patients' medical information to health workers, especially in accident or emergency conditions.
- Patients' manual data entry is reduced, allowing medical staff to watch their patients more effectively.

The organization of the remainder of the chapter is as given: Section 7.2 covers the various works carried out by the researchers in the field of IoT healthcare. Section 7.3 describes the applicability of the Non-conventional health monitors. Section 7.4 describes remote health monitoring including various wearable and non-wearable devices and their applications from the perspective of patients, physicians and the hospital management. Section 7.5 covers the issue of security challenges. Section 7.6 gives an instance of non-conventional health monitors. Section 7.7 concludes the review on this chapter.

7.2 OBJECTIVES OF HEALTHCARE SYSTEMS

By integrating IoT in healthcare, it was witnessed that not only the patient but also the doctor and hospital acquired gains such as, clinical decision making has been improved, minimized replication of analytical testing, imaging, and history taking, preemptive cure, quicker disease diagnosis, medication and equipment supervision, cost reduction, improved patient/doctor collaboration and reduced hospital stays.

Before the advent of non-conventional IoT-based health monitors, the conventional method consisted of visiting doctors and physicians in person and having to move to the hospitals for various checkups and tests for the diagnosis of the disease. This was a very lengthy process, and even involved long hospital stays and even delays in the diagnosis and treatment in such a way that sometimes it used to get very late for the patients to get even cured. Also there was no provision of real-time continuous health monitoring of the patients by the doctor. Patients used to get diagnosed for the duration of their stay in the hospital, but no monitoring afterwards. And patients used to visit hospitals only after observation of serious symptoms which often used to get very late. Although these conventional methods are still in practice, due to unawareness among some sections of the population, the arrival of non-conventional methods has been successful in alleviating the plight of the patients and providing easy and non-delayed monitoring and treatment by the clinicians.

7.3   NON-CONVENTIONAL HEALTH MONITORS

A non-conventional health monitor system is an extension of the medical system of a hospital where a patient's vital body state can be observed distantly. Uninterrupted developments in the semiconductor technology industry have led to sensors and microcontrollers that are smaller in size, quicker in operation, short in power intake and reasonable in cost. With the arrival of sensor and IoT technology, the non-conventional health monitor has become easier to use. Wireless sensors are used to amass and convey signals of interest and a processor is automated to receive and automatically examine the sensor signals.

Nowadays there are many healthcare appliances available in the market which is being frequently used by patients to regularly monitor their health parameters. All these health appliances have different kinds of sensor embedded in them. Electrical, optical, thermal, chemical and other signals can be detected with these sensors, which include transducers [7].

Patient circumstances can be monitored throughout the day by wearable gadgets and non-wearable gadgets with integrated sensors, which can then be reported to the doctor. Non-conventional health monitor system will be an aid in terms of:

- Aids deprived rural people to reach out for the doctor so that suitable direction can be taken and hence lessen the mortality rate in remote areas.
- Minimize overall travel and healthcare costs.
- Medical professionals having real-time access to data boosts the application's potential.
- IoT healthcare applications requirement at any moment and everywhere access.
- Announcement system to doctors in an emergency or if the patient fails to take his or her medication on a regular basis.

As agreed by several people, the internet has changed the world. Ultimately IoT will let patients and service providers work jointly for more productive chronic disease management, more open communication and deeper contribution.

7.4 REMOTE HEALTH MONITORING

Thirty percent of patients re-admit into the hospital after surgery. The cause can be the scarcity of resources for watching patients. It's still a bottleneck to deal with a crisis. With the help of IoT, remote patient monitoring is a possibility. Wearable and non-wearable gadgets with assimilated sensors may monitor and report on a patient's condition throughout the day. With the use of IoT-based remote health monitoring system it would be an aid in terms of:

- Aids deprived rural people to reach out for the doctor so that appropriate direction can be taken and hence reduce the number of deaths in remote locations.
- Lower overall travel and healthcare costs.
- Medical personnel having real-time access to data boosts the application's potential.
- These sorts of IoT solutions are in high demand in healthcare because they may be accessible from anywhere at any time.
- Alerts doctors in the event of an emergency or if a patient fails to take their medication on a regular basis.

As agreed by several people, the internet has changed the world. IoT will eventually allow patients and service providers to work collectively for more fruitful chronic disease management, deeper involvement, and more open communication.

7.4.1 FOR PATIENTS

As the need for healthcare increases speedily, outdated analysis services have not converted enough. With the hasty growing of the ageing population, together with a lengthier life span, E health is set to offer little expenditure and daily domestic practice [1]. In fact, the Remote Mobile Health Monitoring (RMHM) scheme has grown into a study in current time. By making use of the wearable physiologic detection and non-wearable equipment, it is thinkable to observe the consumer's health situation in present time. Also, long-term and uninterrupted discovery is also feasible. As it may aid clinicians, device consistent intensive care and far-flung identification on time [2, 3], RMHM will upgrade the patient's quality of life while also reducing the burden on the medical system and public health spending [4, 5].

7.4.1.1 Wearables

IoT has had a noteworthy influence on the medical field. In recent years, medical IoT wearables have speedily risen to the fore. Right from diagnostics and monitoring to medical methods, the IoT has ensured to provide entirely functional applications which were once only abstract in nature. These IoT wearables shall alter the look of human health care.

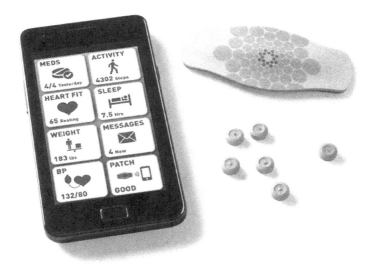

FIGURE 7.1   Ingestible sensor.

Wearable sensors can be well-defined as sensors that are small and sturdy which can be embedded directly on a person's body, such as a wristband or jewellery, or assembled into a smartphone. They are often used to collect data on environmental, physiological, activity, and location variables. Notwithstanding design, wearable sensors gather data for one or more variables (as stated above) and proactively aid in diagnosis and monitoring the health. In the following sub section a few wearables have been explained.

Ingestible Sensors

The ingestible sensor is a sensor-based device that may be taken as a pill. A swallowable sensor is one of the fascinating features of the Internet of Things as shown in Figure 7.1. It discloses a whole new world of potentials of remotely monitoring patients. The ingestible sensors can be utilized to adapt medicines more accurately to reveal each of our medication-taking patterns and lifestyle choices.

One of the best examples is Proteus Digital health, it includes an ingestible sensor with the dimensions of a grain of sand, a tiny wearable sensor patch, a mobile application, and a provider portal. The patient triggers Proteus discovery by using an ingestible sensor to provide medicine. The ingestible sensor sends a signal to the torso patch once it enters the abdomen. A digital record is delivered to the patient's mobile device and subsequently to the Proteus cloud, where healthcare practitioners and caregivers can obtain it via their portal with the patient's consent. The patch also monitors and reports on the patient's activity and so on.

Biosport Hearable Device

This encompasses a wider range of tracking fitness parameters and biometric information through simple ear buds. It aids to track vitals such as heart rate and blood pressure with other important internal aspects, as shown in Figure 7.2.

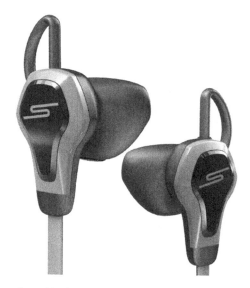

FIGURE 7.2 Biosport hearable device.

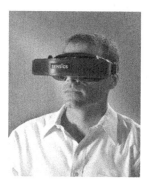

FIGURE 7.3 Smart glass.

Smart Glasses

Smart glass is fundamentally a nursing technology such as artificial intelligence, utilized to clarify vision. A headset is attached on a lens and with the aid of an HD camera, the real-time footage is transmitted on an LED screen. A separate headset device aids the user to enlarge the image and gain the best probable picture. Based on this picture, wearers will give audio commands that will let the navigator direct and steer away from impediments, as shown in Figure 7.3.

Moodables

Moodables promises to enhance relaxation to aid people with trauma disorders. These devices can recognize the brainwaves and transmit low-intensity currents to the brain

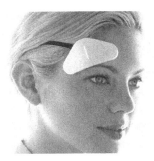

FIGURE 7.4 Moodables.

consequently. These techniques can be utilized on a fit and also on an impaired brain. This will expose a novel branch of study and it can aid to understand a lot about human brain operation and how mood can be elevated, as shown in Figure 7.4.

Smart Watches

Smart watches with disease-specific functions are on the rise, which can be customized as per health monitoring needs. Information collected by the smart watches is synched with apps which either examine or send parameters to a platform for analysis by an HCP (Healthcare Personnel) or caregiver. The biggest progress for smart watches in the health arena is cardiovascular indications.

Fitness Trackers

The fitness tracker are best suited for sports people, stunt lovers and other health cognizant individuals. Fitness trackers are offered as digital connectivity devices and are utilized as an alternative to wristwatches since they give exact fitness-related parameters and encourage a healthy lifestyle. Many sensors are included into fitness trackers to measure mileage, track calorie expenditure, and monitor heart rate and sleep patterns. Fitness trackers are increasing into more user-friendly devices.

Skin Patches

Skin patches are skinny, flexible, adhesive patches including electronic systems that stick onto the skin. They can be either battery or non- battery powered, reusable or not reusable, and give data such as the user's blood pH, sweat rate, and blood chemistry containing ranks of chloride, glucose, lactate, and more. Easy and faster health issue monitoring can be done by wearing of skin patches.

7.4.1.2   Non-Wearables

Along with the wearables, several non-wearable devices such as in commode, bathtub and divan without addition of any biological sensors have been developed for the diagnosis and clinical evaluation of the patients. We are in need of regular one-to-one care of health situations even at our residence for on time and early detection, cure, and prevention of lifestyle-related disarrays, such as adiposis, diabetes, and cardio-vascular disease.

The concept of a smart home came into existence by the use of sensors/devices of many sorts that are incorporated into daily things. The smart home is linked via network technologies in order to collect associated data, such as vital signs and behavioural data, via sensors. These smart homes can be of major help for elderly observation. Also, several other sensors such as motion, radar, object pressure, and ground vibration sensors are used for old health and behaviour observing. Several such ambient sensors are also used for various types of monitoring. Some of them are as follows:

Passive Infrared (PIR) Motion Sensors

The PIR motion sensor is used to perceive the activities of folks. These sensors are mounted on walls or top of the homes to constantly gather signal information that are associated with preset motions inside the sensor's range. PIR motion sensors are generally thermal-sensitive. The sensors sense the existence of people in places by making use of the variation in temperature. PIR motion sensors are utilized at various places to find out transformed kinds of events, for example, hotplate use, apartment temperature, water utilization, location of the user, time spent away from home, sleeping habits, cabinet openings, and night time activities. A base station collects motion data and transmits it to the user's care takers. Then, the collected records are examined for tendencies to find out the variations in daily movements. They can also be examined to find out possible variations in health status.

Video Sensors

Video sensors are one of the most extensively utilised environmental sensors for elder care. These are utilised to track down inhabitants and recognise what they're doing in their houses. Background removal, body form extraction, feature analysis, and machine learning are used to detect movement on walls or ceilings.

Pressure Sensors

The presence of individuals on seats or beds is detected using pressure sensors. They're useful for determining sit-to-stand and stand-to-sit movements.

Sound Sensors

Sensors, such as microphones, are employed to sense a wide range of activities, like the sound created when washing dishes or if an object or person falls.

Floor Sensors

Floor sensors normally looks like a traditional floor and are generally used for both public and private environments. These are used to confirm the location of people so that the lighting and heating systems may be controlled automatically. Floor sensors are employed in the majority of smart eldercare systems to detect emergency situations such as falls. During public events, they may also be used to count people and observe crowd movements.

7.4.2 FOR PHYSICIANS

With the use of IoT-based health wearable and non-wearable devices, clinician can observe patients' health more efficiently. Information collected from IoT devices can aid clinicians find out the best suited treatment for patients and achieve the desired results. It helps clinicians to make evidence-based decisions while also ensuring openness. Consistent patient observation and real-time data aids in analysing diseases as soon as possible.

7.4.2.1 Healthcare Charting

The example of these IoT devices includes Audemix which is commanded by voice in order to generate the readily accessible data of the patient which can be quickly accessed by the doctors, hence saving the time and effort of both the doctor and patients.

7.4.2.2 Wireless Patient Monitoring

This application is a proven boon for sharing distant observation real-time data between patients and doctors from varied locations. Chronic disease management, such as hypertension, diabetes, coronary heart disease and asthma, is made easier using such applications. Wirelessly monitored pacemakers and automated defibrillators are two such examples.

7.4.2.3 Virtual Consultation (Telemedicine)

Virtual care consultations, education, medicine distribution and therapeutic procedures are all part of this application. These applications are useful in avoiding booking appointments and waiting times. Via virtualization, this problem can be addressed within minutes and even seconds. The use of robots and nursing aides in tele surgery for regular procedures appears to be feasible.

7.4.2.4 Aging in Place

Such type of applications are used to take care of elderly aged population. These applications includes wearables which continuously monitor the plight of these people and sends the information to the care takers. The information may be utilized to provide medical assistance to those in need, and in the event of more serious irregularities, the closest efficient hospitals can be notified, reducing hospitalisation costs by early intervention and treatment. Examples include personal emergency responses systems (PERS), video sessions and movement observation and fall detection.

7.4.2.5 VSee Team

It is a real-time telemedicine eye clinic. This telemedicine package includes all of the fundamental healthcare diagnostic gadgets (stethoscope, heart rate, blood pressure, pulse oximeter, ultrasounds, otoscopes, dermascopes and so on) that are linked to the doctor remotely. It is as shown in Figure 7.3. All such devices send the real-time information to the doctor through video conference. Such kits can be comfortably utilized and operated by the technicians with a meagre experience and training.

7.4.3 FOR HOSPITALS

Not only are IoT devices used for handling patients and facilitating clinicians, these devices find a vital application in hospital management as well. These devices, when mounted with sensors, facilitate in locating medical equipment such as wheelchairs, defibrillators, nebulizers, oxygen pumps and other surveillance systems in real-time. Medical personnel's duties at various positions can also be analysed in real-time.

IoT-enabled hygiene monitoring devices are useful for preventing the spread of illnesses in hospitals. They also help with asset management, such as pharmaceutical inventories control and atmospheric surveillance, such as checking the temperature and humidity of the refrigerator, treatment compliance monitoring, supported living, smarter medication, and telemedicine. IoT sensors can be mounted on several pieces of medical equipment like wheelchairs, defibrillators, nebulizers and oxygen pumps so that assets may be managed effectively. Administration of medicines and health apparatuses has been a main bottleneck in a healthcare application. By making use of the IoT, these are managed and utilized efficiently with minimized expenditure.

7.4.3.1 Device Monitoring

In order to accomplish device monitoring, an IoT embedded device notifies when it notices any malfunctioning in the device.

7.4.3.2 Asset Management in Hospitals

Hospital inventory management is of vital importance for various reasons including demand forecasting, managing the expenses if the hospital under control and as per regulations decided by the hospital management, to make choices regarding the store stock in accordance with the ongoing inflow and outflow of patients. A disruption in resources can endanger the patients' lives and health medical inventory management relies heavily on forecasting. The scarcity of visibility and incorporation of already-present data, i.e. data that is routinely collected but kept in various information systems, into fruitful demand forecasting that can aid in improving medical inventory management, is one of the key issues that hospital managers are concerned about.

During the construction of the IoT facilitated hospital, sensors are mounted at different locations for the purpose of management.

7.4.3.3 Environment Management

Sensors installed on the buildings during construction, gives data pertaining to the air quality, temperature, humidity, light level, earthquake recognition, etc. on which additional processing is carried out to retrieve meaningful facts.

7.4.3.4 Smart Wheelchairs and Stretchers

These smart IoT devices are found at different locations of the hospital. These help in deciding the necessary and required treatment of the injured patients. This not only saves the time of the clinician from testing, but facilitates ease of treatment. In order to observe the activities of the patients within the span of area, smart wheelchairs are also often used.

7.4.3.5 WBLC

The purpose of wireless building lighting control is to alter the light intensity in the room for the patient's comfort and for power saving.

7.4.3.6 Swasthya Slate

Swasthya is a Sanskrit word that denotes "health, soundness, and well-being." Swasthya slate is used to perform the fundamental tests. It gives immediate findings and guidance, allowing for more effective and efficient therapy.

7.4.3.7 Information System

The patient's admittance, enrollment, expenditures, patient care maintenance and report management are all handled through an information system.

7.4.3.8 Smart Beds and Washable Clothing

Smart beds and washable smart clothes are used to monitor patients who are admitted to the hospital. An alarm is sent out if the patient's health requires care, and doctors are summoned to assess them.

7.5 SECURITY CHALLENGES

Traditional security techniques are less helpful to fulfil the security necessities of the IoT devices. Thus, in order to ensure the security, the IoT devices have to face novel security bottlenecks. A collection of characteristics for IoT security may be found in the given things.

7.5.1 COMPUTATIONAL LIMITATIONS

All IoT health devices face computational limitations since they have low speed processors which are not powerful, they perform simple tasks, hence do not support complex and expensive operations. They are just simple sensors or actuators. Thus, the major challenging bottlenecks that disturb the IoT devices are achieving the maximal performance in terms of security with the minimal consumptions of the resources.

7.5.2 MEMORY LIMITATIONS

IoT healthcare devices have limits since they possess low memory. In order to trigger such devices, there is need of an fixed operating system (OS), system software and an application. Hence, their recall isn't up to the task of implementing complicated security procedures.

7.5.3 ENERGY LIMITATIONS

In addition to memory constraints, IoT healthcare devices have a limited battery life (e.g. body temperature and BP sensors). When not in use, these IoT systems conserve energy by switching to a power-saving mode.

7.5.4   MOBILITY

Basically, healthcare devices are not static, they move from place to place as a person moves. IoT service providers link these devices to the internet. Thus, in order to be in range of IoT service provider, these devices have to lie in a predefined range of area.

7.5.5   SCALABILITY

As the number of IoT appliances grows, so does the number of devices linked to the internet; thus, designing a secure scalable system is a big challenge for researchers.

7.5.6   COMMUNICATION MEDIA

IoT fitness systems are connected to either native or worldwide or both systems via various wireless networks like Zigbee, Z-Wave, Bluetooth, Bluetooth Low Energy, WiFi, GSM, WiMax and 3G/4G. The conventional security schemes that are applicable to wired channels cannot be applied to wireless channel features of these networks. Hence, it is a tedious task to discover and use a general security mechanism that can be consistently applied to both connectivity wired and wireless channel elements.

7.5.7   THE MULTIPLICITY OF DEVICES

IoT Health appliances have a wide range of variety encompassing the personal computers to little-end RFID tags. These devices keep on changing by their computational, power, memory limitations as well as the software embedded into them. Thus, such a security mechanism that can accommodate all types of IoT healthcare devices, even the simplest one, is still a bottleneck that has to be addressed.

7.5.8   A DYNAMIC TOPOLOGY

The anywhere and anytime availability feature of the healthcare network based on the Internet of Things gives birth to the need of adapting new topology wherever required, hence the need for dynamic topology is encouraged.

7.5.9   A MULTI-PROTOCOL NETWORK

A health device might need to interconnect with other devices either lying in the native or in the global network supporting different and non-uniform protocols. Hence these devices should be designed to accommodate this feature.

7.5.10   DATA CONFIDENTIALITY

In order to maintain the integrity and the confidentiality of the medical sensitive data, it's still a challenge to build such mechanisms.

7.5.11 TRUST MECHANISMS

A faith negotiating system, arbitration language, or object identity management system must be used to sustain communication between peers.

7.6 TECHNOLOGIES USED FOR AN IOT HEALTHCARE SYSTEM

The current two technologies that are often used to support remote health monitoring system are: cloud computing and fog computing.

7.6.1 CLOUD COMPUTING FOR HEALTHCARE

Cloud computing has proved to be the most promising technology for IoT healthcare systems. By offering desired computing capabilities (e.g. storage, service, networks, servers, applications and hardware) to users, cloud computing provides scalability, mobility, and security benefits. Various research revealed that cloud computing is the backbone for supporting IoT healthcare system.

7.6.2 FOG COMPUTING ARCHITECTURE

Fog computing is a virtualized platform that connects end devices to the cloud for processing, storing, and networking. The rudimentary idea behind fog computing is to move data centre tasks to fog nodes located somewhere at the network's edge. The fog layer is what we call these fog nodes. Because the gadgets that conduct the activities are all at the network's edge, they have a faster data transmission rate and a faster user response time.

Fog computing can be most beneficial in applications that require a large volume of information to be analysed in a short interval of time and that's the reason advancement in remote health monitoring will be easier and more efficient. Applications in healthcare system: this is a sector where instantaneous processing is crucial. Hence, the data should be processed quickly and the reaction time must be as short as feasible.

For this, a fog layer will improve healthcare observation delay and enable real-time health monitoring. By the presence of this layer, security is also ensured and third party manipulation of data is also circumvented for the patients' details.

Table 7.1 analyses and contrasts the many properties of cloud and fog computing. The fog-assisted system may improve scalability, energy awareness, mobility, and reliability in IoT healthcare systems.

Figure 7.5 shows overall healthcare concept and application.

7.7 CONCLUSION

Earlier, before the advent of non-conventional IoT-based health monitors, the conventional method consisted of visiting to the doctors and physicians in person and to move to the hospitals for various checkups and tests for the diagnosis of the disease. This was a very lengthy process, and even involved long hospital stays and even delay

TABLE 7.1
Several Aspects of Cloud Computing and Fog Computing Are Compared

Characteristics	Cloud Computing	Fog Computing
Node location	The internet	Local network edge
Number of node	Little	Large
Latency	High	Low
Delay	High	Low
Distance between devices and server	Multiple hops	Single hop
Location awareness	No	No
Distribution	Centralized	Distributed
Scalability	Supported (dynamic adaptation workload)	Limited (fog is not as scalable as cloud)
Mobility support	Limited	Good
Real-time interaction	Supported	Supported
Data storage	Huge	Limit
Transmission	Device to cloud	Device to device
Data aggregation	At cloud	Partially and remaining to cloud
Security	No user-defined security (carried out by cloud service providers)	User-defined security (data is processed by a complex distributed system)

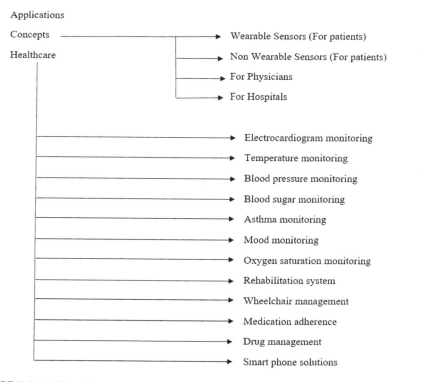

FIGURE 7.5   IoT healthcare concepts and applications.

in the diagnosis and treatment in such a way that sometimes it used to get very late for the patients to get even cured. Also there was no provision of real-time continuous health monitoring of the patients by the doctor. Patients used to get diagnosed for the duration they stay in the hospital, but no monitoring afterwards. And patients used to visit hospitals only after observation of serious symptoms which often used to get very late. Although these conventional methods are still in practice due to unawareness among some sections of the population, the arrival of nonconventional methods has been successful in alleviating the plight of the patients and easy and non-delayed monitoring and treatment by the clinicians.

REFERENCES

1. Tamilselvi V, Sribalaji S, Vigneshwaran P, Vinu P, GeethaRamani J. IoT based health monitoring system. In: 2020 6th International conference on advanced computing and communication systems (ICACCS). IEEE; 2020: 386–9.
2. Acharya AD, Patil SN. IoT based health care monitoring kit. In: 2020 Fourth international conference on computing methodologies and communication (ICCMC). IEEE; 2020: 363–8.
3. Banerjee S, Roy S. Design of a photo plethysmography based pulse rate detector. Int J Rec Trends Eng Res. 2016; 2: 302–6.
4. M. Haghi et al., A flexible and pervasive IoT-based healthcare platform for physiological and environmental parameters monitoring. IEEE Internet of Things Journal. 2020; 7, 6: 5628–5647.
5. Shubham Banka, Isha Madan and S.S. Saranya, Smart healthcare monitoring using IoT. International Journal of Applied Engineering Research. 2018; 13, 15: 11984–11989.
6. S. Trivedi and A. N. Cheeran, Android based health parameter monitoring. 2017 International Conference on Intelligent Computing and Control Systems (ICICCS), Madurai, India, 2017: 1145–1149.
7. B. Xu, L. D. Xu, H. Cai, C. Xie, J. Hu, and F. Bu. Ubiquitous data accessing method in IoT-based information system for emergency medical services. IEEE Transactions on Industrial Informatics. 2014; 10, 2:1578–1586.
8. Gregoski MJ, Mueller M, Vertegel A, Shaporev A, Jackson BB, Frenzel RM, Sprehn SM, Treiber FA. Development and validation of a smartphone heart rate acquisition application for health promotion and wellness telehealth applications. Int J Telemed Appl. 2012: 1–7.
9. Oresko JJ, Jin Zhanpeng, Cheng Jun, Huang Shimeng, Sun Yuwen, Duschl H, Cheng AC. A wearable smartphone-based platform for real-time cardiovascular disease detection via electrocardiogram processing. IEEE Tran INF Technol Biomed. 2010; 14: 734–40.
10. Islam, M.M., Rahaman, A. & Islam, M.R. Development of smart healthcare monitoring system in IoT environment. SN Comput. Sci. 2020; 1: 185.
11. www.pcworld.com/article/2898129/sms-audio-biosport-earbuds-review-heart-rate-monitoring-headphones-are-more-convenient-than-you-thi.html.
12. www.heypayless.com/5-iot-applications-that-will-change-the-face-of-healthcare/.
13. H. Hafezi, T. L. Robertson, G. D. Moon, K. Au-Yeung, M. J. Zdeblick and G. M. Savage, An Ingestible Sensor for Measuring Medication Adherence. IEEE Transactions on Biomedical Engineering. 2015; 62, 1: 99–109.

14. F. John Dian, R. Vahidnia and A. Rahmati, Wearables and the Internet of Things (IoT), Applications, Opportunities, and Challenges: A Survey. IEEE Access. 2020; 8: 69200–69211.

15. Md. Zia Uddin, Weria Khaksar and Jim Torresen, Ambient sensors for elderly care and independent living: A Survey, MDPI, 2018.

16. https://vsee.com/blog/syrian-refugees-vsee-telemedicine-duhok/.

17. www.mobihealthnews.com/content/senseonics-launches-norway-completes-fda-premarket-submission.

18. https://infobionic.com/cardiac-monitoring-solution-how-it-works/.

19. www.wipro.com/business-process/what-can-iot-do-for-healthcare.

20. www.iot-now.com/2019/09/27/99050-regulation-reimbursement-strategies-not-get-way-smart-electronic-skin-patches/.

8 Applications, Opportunities, and Current Challenges in the Healthcare Industry

Veena A. and Gowrishankar S.
Dr. Ambedkar Institute of Technology, Bengaluru, India

CONTENTS

8.1 INTRODUCTION

Healthcare is the maintenance or improvement of a person's health through the prevention, diagnosis, treatment, recovery, or cure of disease, illness, injury, and other physical and mental disabilities. Wellness and health are important aspects of our lives that influence our quality of life. Given increasingly limited economic resources, efficient delivery of quality healthcare is a critical societal goal [1]. In the medical field, we collect large amounts of data on individuals and their medical problems through medical registries and many other medical procedures [2]. Healthcare organizations are transitioning from paper-based records to electronic records. Using electronic health records and other forms of automation has transformed the healthcare industry

DOI: 10.1201/9781003145035-8

[3]. Instant access to genuine patient information from anywhere in the globe has brought prospective benefits that cannot be accessed by the widespread usage of digital data in healthcare. Electronic healthcare records (EHR) have replaced traditional paper-based records. With the rapid growth of electronic gadgets and greater internet access, more devices are now linked to the internet than individuals. The healthcare industry, which has been sluggish to accept new technology, is predicted to have over 80 million linked devices by 2022, despite its slow adoption rate. In addition, different health application areas represent different opportunities for IoT adoption and, according to current trends, application areas of smart health products (for example, smart drugs, smart dispensers and syringes, smart device monitoring, lockers Smart RFID, Electronic Health Records, etc.) are the hottest [4].

Data sources in the healthcare industry include the human generated data, biometric data, machine-generated data, behavioural data, epidemiological data, transactional data and publication data [5]. Health monitoring in non-hospital settings, particularly at home, has long piqued the interest of healthcare researchers and developers. Continuous monitoring of physiological data in daily life, such as ECG signals or heart rate, is critical for controlling chronic conditions, such as cardiovascular disease [6]. Big data is a next-generation technology and architecture designed to economically derive value from vast amounts of types of data by enabling fast collection, detection and analysis [7]. In the healthcare context, big data refers to a large and complex collection of electronic health data that is difficult to process, distribute, and analyse using standard approaches and methods.

We expect health data analysis to have a significant impact on current treatments as life expectancy increases with the global population. Health analysis can help predict epidemics, reduce treatment costs, prevent preventable diseases and improve the quality of care and the lives of patients. Data analytics in healthcare can make it simpler to collect medical data and turn it into meaningful insights that can then be utilised to improve care. For healthcare applications, enormous patient data contain valuable and significant insights that can be exposed through data analysis employing modern machine learning, deep learning and data mining algorithms [8].

In a cloud computing environment, we may examine healthcare data to solve a diversity of challenges in the healthcare industry [9]. Cloud computing inherits the capabilities of high-performance parallel computing, grid computing, and distributed computing, and evolves these methods to achieve location transparency and improve the user experience on the internet [10]. The use of cloud computing technologies is excellent for healthcare facilities because of its on-demand services, high scalability, and virtualization capabilities. Many articles now report on the combination of cloud and health, and some articles call it the e-health cloud [11].

For medical data management, we can use cloud computing in the healthcare domain. If an outbreak is suspected, each healthcare provider has access to or hosts a cloud platform that may store, process, and distribute data among patients, healthcare workers and other stakeholders (such as centers for disease control and prevention if an outbreak is detected). A platform of this type can also house services for managing the identities of all patient consent, registered users and patient health data and reports. The cloud platform may also help the healthcare professionals with administrative activities, such as updating and generating billing reports and disbursing payments.

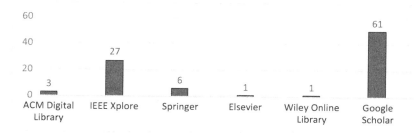

FIGURE 8.1   Database sources for healthcare domain research articles.

Public and private cloud infrastructure used by multiple healthcare providers can integrate using a cross-cloud architecture to communicate patient data, create billing profiles, and more to meet patient mobility needs [12].

Because the cloud cannot address all the quality of service (QoS) needs of IoT and the technological revolution it brings, introducing of fog computing is a win-win opportunity for a variety of sectors such as body area networks (BANs), healthcare, vehicle networks, and smart grids [13]. The goal of fog-based architecture is to handle the processing and streaming of data from a variety of healthcare devices and equipment. Moving the processing of healthcare data streams closer to the data sources at the edge can minimize network traffic and improve the latency of time-sensitive healthcare applications. Typical fog data streams processing components includes a data stream processing engine, distributed messaging system and data storage. The architecture's fog computer layer is based on the popular Apache Kafka's sophisticated message system and the influential Apache Storm workflow appliance that handles large amounts of data [14].

As shown in Figure 8.1, we performed the search across different online databases identifying sample papers between 2010 and 2021.

We organized the rest of the chapter as follows. Section 8.2 highlights the different types of healthcare data generated from various devices. We discussed many research problems and issues in healthcare that originate from various entities in Section 8.3. Section 8.4 covers the use of the blockchain technology in the healthcare industry and Section 8.5 covers healthcare analytics. A thorough examination of the major contributions of IoT and cloud-based mechanisms in medical applications is covered in Section 8.6 and Section 8.7 and 8.8 covers the security and privacy, and conclusion respectively.

8.2   HEALTHCARE DATA

Healthcare is considered a data-intensive sector [15]. The traditional process for capturing critical patient data is labour intensive for collecting, entering, and analysing information. These processes are often slow and error-prone, causing delays in accessibility of the real-time data [12]. With so many patients and little time, there is an urgent need to develop a new and scalable big data infrastructure and analytical methods that enable healthcare practitioners to access knowledge for each particular person. This requires a framework that uses patient EHRs and genetics data to facilitate predictive, personalized, preventative and participative healthcare decision making.

Advances in information technology have made it easier to access large amounts of health data, such as electronic health records (EHR). Medical history, demographics, prescription, lab test results and billing information are all included in EHR data [16]. Operational databases, transactional databases, domain-specific databases, knowledge bases, temporary caches, memory grids, big data stores and other data stores are all examples of data storages. Financial and operational databases, and electronic health records (EHR) of hospitals and clinics, Genome database, database of insurance pharmaceutical firms, knowledge bases, drug research data, ontologies unique to healthcare and other important data are available in the healthcare domain. Data can be extracted and analysed from any of these forms of data storage, depending on the analytical requirements [17].

Most health and medical research relies on clinical data. Clinical data is collected either as part of an ongoing or as part of a formal clinical study programme. We can divide clinical data into six prime categories: administrative data, claims data, electronic health records, patient, illness, disease enrolment, clinical trials data and health surveys. The registry is patient-centred, goal-based and designed to extract information about identified health and exposure outcomes [18].

Access to high-quality health data is an important requirement for healthcare professionals and pharmaceuticals researchers to make informed decisions. According to [19], health data can be divided into four groups: data from medical insurance (data acquired and held by several health insurance organizations for several years), clinical data (records for patient health, operational and laboratory reports and medical images, etc.), patient behaviour data (data collected via wearable devices and monitors) and data from drug research (reports on clinical studies, high performance results screening). The various types of healthcare data that contribute to big healthcare data are depicted in Figure 8.2.

Benefits of electronic health records includes higher quality care, more accurate patient information, interoperability, increased efficiency, increased revenue, scalability, accessibility, personalization, security and support. Privacy and security issues are drawbacks of using EHR. Another difficulty is how patients use and comprehend the data on patient portals. It is critical that patients do not misinterpret file entries. Furthermore, staff workers may not use the EHR platform effectively. An EHR system's appropriate implementation could take months or even years. Smaller health centres and more skilled specialists may prefer to do everything on paper, but others do not, which can lead to misunderstanding. At first, implementing EHR may seem to slow things down, but once the learning curve is overcome, the benefits far outweigh.

8.3 HEALTHCARE RESEARCH ISSUES

Many issues in healthcare stem from the complicated network of middlemen and the failure to trace the transactions. Healthcare data is broken down into multiple silos which have detrimental impacts on research and services [20].

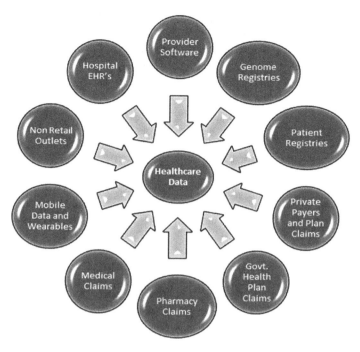

FIGURE 8.2 Different types of healthcare data.

1. In the healthcare system, there are several technical challenges in research and clinical procedures [21].
   a. **Policy making**: The healthcare system requires interoperability between private and public stakeholders. This emphasises the need for nationally / internationally coordinated standards and agreements that span boundaries and authorities.
   b. **Lack of regulation**: The development of relevant rules for governance of proprietary rights of ownership related to clinical transactions for the envisaged healthcare system is proving problematic across the world. Because there are so many parties, data ownership and current health law in the traditional healthcare system are critical concerns that must be addressed. It will be difficult to change the present regulatory structure to meet new administration policy objectives controlling digitally defined, computerized and ubiquitous nature. The ownership of healthcare data, permitted access privileges, distributed storage structure should all be well defined.
   c. **Confidentiality and transparency**: in certain situations, technology emphasises transparency, which may be undesirable in the healthcare realm. Although it provides security through encryption, healthcare stakeholders consider the accessibility of a database, even in encrypted

form, to be a significant concern. As a result, adequate access control should be addressed in healthcare informatics [22].

d. **Sustainability**: In healthcare informatics systems, the encryption key is very essential. The private encryption key cannot be recovered. Because of its long-term nature, this increases the difficulty of healthcare data. The trustworthiness and utility of a patient's health record are reduced when parts of them are missing. In addition, hacking or robbing the private key of a user gives access to all user-specified information.

e. **Manageability of data**: Healthcare systems expand when users add data. Because of the increased computational power and storage needs, the network may have fewer edge nodes with sufficient processing capacity to analyse and evaluate data in the Healthcare systems. When healthcare practitioners cannot fulfil the needs of storage and computer capacity, the possibility for more centralization and delayed validation and confirmation of data increases.

f. **Adoption of new technologies**: In the health industry, new technologies, such as blockchain and Artificial Intelligence, are gaining popularity. Blockchain and cloud computing of both technologies rely on a network of interconnected computers to provide computational power. We must reward contributors for donating computer power through incentive mechanisms. Health organizations may require encouragement to embrace new technologies.

g. **Operating cost**: The cost of setting up and running the healthcare system, and the cost of migrating from existing health informatics system, is unknown, open-source technology and the intermittent nature of the technology can assist operating cost. The ongoing operation and maintenance of the health informatics system demands continuous availability of trouble-solving, updating, backup and reporting resources.

2. Several approaches to the detection of falls have been presented during the last two decades. Because of the rapid development of new technologies, this problem is quite active in the scientific community. Although significant progress has been achieved, there are still several difficulties to overcome [23].

a. The scarcity of real-world data: there is no standard public dataset available. There are many simulated data sets by individual sensors accessible, but it is questionable whether models based on data gathered by young and healthy individuals can apply to older persons in real-life settings. There is a need to develop a benchmark data set consisting of data from many sensors.

b. Real-time detection: researchers need to focus more on real-time systems that can be used in the actual world. Security and privacy must be addressed in tandem with fall detection systems.

c. Platform of sensor fusion: comprehensive research is required to build entire information systems capable of dealing with data management and transmission in an efficient, effective, and secure manner in order to bring solutions closer to the market.

    d. Locational constraint: sensors are permanent and static, such as visual ones. Fall detection systems that can be used in both regulated and uncontrolled situations are required.

    e. Scalability and flexibility: with the rising number of affordable sensors, the scalability of fall detection systems must be investigated, when considering heterogeneous sensors [24].

3. Despite AI's claimed accomplishments in cancer imaging, there are several limitations and roadblocks to overcome before widespread clinical usage [25].

    a. Medical imaging data is seldom curated for labelling, quality assurance, annotations, segmentation, or suitability for the task at hand. Medical data interpretation is a key roadblock in the development of automated healthcare solutions since it causes the employment of trained experts, making the process time and expense intensive. In the medical field, standardised benchmarking is especially important, given the wide range of imaging techniques and anatomic locations, as well as gathering standards and hardware.

    b. Interpretability and integrity of AI: The value of trust and openness in AI systems is differentiated according to their performance, which makes it possible to identify defects when AI is subhuman and therefore transform superhuman AI into a future educator. Complex evaluations of biological networks may have a significant influence on response and prognosis assessment, as well as therapy planning, with the integration of AI.

    c. Imaging is not a stand-alone indicator of illness. It is becoming abundantly clear that cancer genetic fingerprints, such as non-invasive blood biomarkers of tumour, socio-economic position and even social networks, have an influence on the fate of cancer individuals.

8.4 HEALTHCARE BLOCKCHAIN SYSTEMS

Because of its advanced characteristics such as traceability, security and transparency, blockchain (BC) has become one of the most popular technologies in the internet era [26]. Blockchain technology allows for the storage of information in such a way that it is nearly difficult to add, remove or change the information without being discovered by other operatives [27]. As one of the most fascinating technical breakthroughs, blockchain technology is fast gaining popularity in the healthcare industry [28]. The instances of effective blockchain healthcare implementations include the Gem Health Network [29], Patientory Inc. (patientory.com/), SimplyVital health, MedRec [30], etc.

Blockchain may be divided into the following categories [31]: Public blockchain, Federated blockchain and Private blockchain. Public blockchain is a permissionless blockchain, so anybody may conduct transactions anonymously or pseudo anonymously. Furthermore, it is an open network with the highest level of decentralised trust. This includes cryptocurrencies such as Bitcoin, Ethereum, Waves[32], Dash[33], and Bitshares [34]. Federated blockchain is a licensed blockchain and works on the initiative of a group called consortium. The transactions might be open to the public or

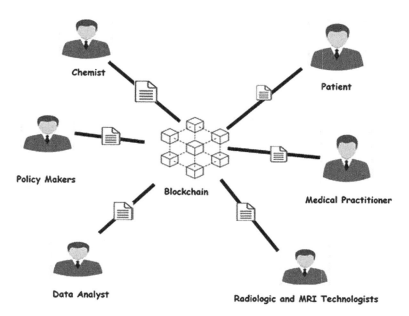

FIGURE 8.3 Blockchain as a platform for healthcare [35].

kept hidden. This category includes EWF (Energy), R3 Corda, and B3i (Insurance). Private blockchain is a permissioned blockchain designed to supervise and validate internal organization transactions. It could be accessible to the general public or not. Blocks are generated more quickly and with a better throughput. The private blockchain is used to assess trustworthiness, which depends on the algorithm used, not on authority. This includes Monax and Hyper Ledger with Sawtooth.

The healthcare sector can benefit from a variety of blockchain systems. Figure 8.3 illustrates the combination of blockchain and IoT technologies that allow healthcare organizations to efficiently and accurately manage records, which is critical. We outline the complete process, beginning with the collection of real-time data from patients via IoT and ending with the provision of a suitable drug that ensures the patient's happiness [35]. The blockchain technology comprises of several interconnected components. Blockchain technology can make certain guarantees to its users by combining these components.

- **Blockchain**: like a traditional ledger, is a digital ledger or an immutable record at its most fundamental level. At the heart of the blockchain is the ledger. This is a recording infrastructure that allows ledger owners to tell a story about the transactions. Although ledgers can store almost any type of data imaginable, this topic usually centres on asset ownership and history [36].
- **Cryptography**: cryptography, or the study of how to convey data in a secure or genuine manner, is another vital component of blockchain technology. Utilization of encryption in blockchain technology to preserve anonymity,

offer ledger immutability and authenticate claims made against assets recorded and controlled on the blockchain. Today to connect a block, the information in the block is being sent to a process called a "cryptographic hash". A cryptographic hash function produces a separate output or ID for a particular input. Depending on inputs, each block's hash will always be unique. When the data in a block changes, the hash or ID generated on the next block in the chain no longer matches the original value. The current block's header carries the hash of the preceding block to connect or chain data blocks together. Changing the contents of any block in a blockchain results in an entirely non-identical hash, and the new hash will not match the hash in the following block header, causing the blockchain to break and invalidate all blocks related to the location of the changes. As a result, blockchain technology is highly censorship-resistant and tamper-resistant [37].

- **Peer-to-peer network**: blockchain heavily relies on current computer networking technologies, particularly peer-to-peer network topologies. Blockchain is built on the same technology that underpins our modern internet's backbone. Using peer-to-peer network design promotes redundancy and fault tolerance by eliminating single points of failure that are frequent in traditional client / server network topologies [38]. Any transaction initiated by any node in the network will be validated by peer nodes. The block will be expanded to include the validated transaction.
- **Assets**: eventually, any blockchain system must include assets. Assets are items which we keep track of, the assets that 'matter' with a specific outcome or use case scenarios. An asset is something that requires a proof of ownership. Healthcare data, event tickets, an auto title or a patent are samples of monetary, non-monetary or informational assets. Blockchain started as a registry system for recording the digital data transfer of digital "tokens" or "coins", such as Bitcoin and other cryptocurrencies.
- **Consensus algorithm**: consensus is a method of ensuring that all connected device validate transactions and agree on their order and presence on the ledger. There are several options that fit different situations when there is agreement. Opportunity cost (security, speed, etc.) is considered when deciding whether or not to utilize a particular consensus mechanism. The major distinction between them is how consensus systems delegate and reward transaction verification. Proof-of-work and proof-of-stake are the most used consensus algorithms.
- **Smart contract**: the software or business logic that runs on the ledger.
- **Affiliation/certificate authority**: to join the network, the user must be granted authorization. The user's identity is verified by the certificate authority and ensures that they have appropriate access to the ledger for the transaction they are executing.

By making substantial improvements, blockchain technology can help streamline data management in healthcare such as improved drug traceability, patient record management, clinical trials and precision medicine, maintaining consistent permissions, protecting healthcare systems, optimizing health insurance coverage and healthcare billing systems. The open research challenges in blockchain in healthcare includes

TABLE 8.1
Blockchain Techniques Used in Healthcare Applications

Blockchain Methods Used	Healthcare Examples	Advantages	Disadvantages
Blockchain private hyperledger fabric [40]	Behavioural health data collected using a mobile phone.	Tamper resistant healthcare platform for behavioral therapy.	Obsolete codes and consensus algorithm.
The Ethereum platform and a consortium-managed blockchain [41]	Remote patient monitoring.	Real-time health information is gained by sensors is managed, monitored, and securely analyzed.	Data transfer is not secure since it uses public network from body sensors to blockchain nodes. As the number of sensors increases, key management will become an issue, verification of the healthcare data is delayed.
Consortium PoW [42]	Pharmaceutical data.	Prevents counterfeit drugs and tracks the flow of drugs.	Cost is high, and investigation of policies and regulations.
Proof of concept with timestamp [43]	Clinical trials, Electronic Health Records (EHR).	Consent in clinical trials and EHR	Concern over security of the data, and whether or not the patient has signed the consent.
Smart contract with permissioned blockchain [44]	Patient and drug dose information	Delivery of drugs in the secure way with prescription and patient information.	The quantity of the users increases the response time and system latency.

scalability, interoperability, navigating regulation uncertainty, tokenization of data, irreversibility and quantum computing, incorporating blockchain technology into established healthcare organizations, ensuring healthcare data accuracy and blockchain developers culture adoption [39]. Table 8.1 compares and contrasts the various Blockchain techniques for the healthcare trade, as well as their benefits and drawbacks.

8.5   HEALTHCARE ANALYTICS

Healthcare analytics is well-defined as the "systematic application of data and related clinical and business (C & B) insights developed through applied analytical disciplines

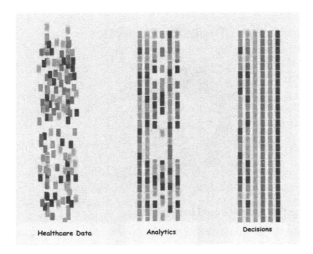

Healthcare Data   Analytics   Decisions

FIGURE 8.4   Healthcare data, analytics and decisions [48].

such as statistical, contextual, quantitative, predictive and cognitive spectrums to drive fact-based decision making for planning, management, measurement and learning" [45,46]. Healthcare data analytics is being used not just for the study of clinical data and electronic health records (EHR), but also for getting insights into related businesses such as pharmaceuticals, healthcare insurance firms, and so on [47]. Figure 8.4 shows the three steps of healthcare analytics [48]. The first step is the data collection. Healthcare comprises of different data such as electronic health records (EHR), medical claims, wearable devices, etc. There are several tools for processing, visualising and analysing data after obtaining the data. Finally, it's time to take a decision. A good understanding of the patient's illness is aided by an analytics report. Big data helps healthcare practitioners to negotiate more efficient operations and information on patients and their health. Big data has several applications in the healthcare sector.

8.5.1 Types of Analytics

Healthcare analytics may be classified into three main types: descriptive, predictive and prescriptive analytics. Figure 8.5 depicts the analytics employed in the literature review.

1. **Descriptive analytics**: descriptive analytics is about investigating the information in the data set. As the name suggests, it is used to characterize large data sets, compressing them into manageable data sets, charts, or statistics that physicians can use. To quantify raw data, descriptive analytics employs both historical and present data. Hospitals, for example, may examine readmissions to get insight into trends that might minimize and boost patient care.
2. **Predictive analytics**: predictive analytics are used to forecast outcomes, such as patient outcomes, depending on the quantity and severity of risk symptoms

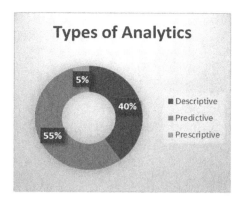

FIGURE 8.5   Types of analytics used in healthcare.

exhibited. This makes use of the same historical data, but in a different way: as a foundation for projecting future events or outcomes. In healthcare, such as population health, this has obvious benefit. A physician, for example, might anticipate chronic disease patterns in rural communities and act.

3. **Prescriptive analytics**: stakeholders can predict more futures based on the precautions taken and analyse how useful each tactic is for other options. Prescriptive analytics can help practitioners in determining which course of action is practical and gives the greatest potential benefit, such as when developing department-wide performance improvement goals as an executive.

Descriptive analytics go back in time to explain what happened and why. Predictive and prescriptive analytics make use of previous data to anticipate what will happen in the near future and what measures to take to influence those results.

8.6   HEALTHCARE APPLICATIONS

All people in today's society are battling in their busy lives to prioritise their health. The extraordinary success of health applications shows that increasing numbers of individuals rely on technology to care for themselves and fulfil their health goals. Cloud computing is being used by healthcare application providers to handle massive processing loads and lower service delivery costs [49]. Personal well-being management necessitates the provision of individualized services via dynamically generated ecosystems [50].

8.6.1   APPLICATIONS FOR PATIENTS

For successful healthcare systems, it is crucial to raise the standard of living and experience of patient's healthcare services. The goals of healthcare applications that serve patients differ; yet, they are related to and complement one another [51]. Using different electronic gadgets and technologies for patient self-management is referred to as telehealth, telemedicine, m-health and e-health.

Telehealth emerged to enable remote patient monitoring and to deliver healthcare services across long distances. The geographical distance between the healthcare practitioner and the patient is bridged [52]. m-health and e-health both play an important role in supporting healthcare with electronic gadgets. They serve the same purpose, but the major distinction is in how the information is delivered. Mobile devices, such as handheld devices, smartphones, personal digital assistants (PDAs) or a tablets are used to assist healthcare practices in m-health. Patients are permitted to use their personal mobile devices to log, save, and monitor their health records via m-health services. These services aid in the improvement of the efficiency with which healthcare information is delivered. The m-health application can be very beneficial for professionals and patients to study and use. The term "e-health" encompasses a much larger knowledge of healthcare procedures which are assisted by integrating technologies.

Telehealth is the transmission of information and healthcare services between healthcare practitioners and patients via telecommunication technologies for patient care and monitoring. To meet the needs of developing countries, telecommunication services necessitate significant infrastructure investment [53]. Primary healthcare professionals in rural areas are frequently separated and secluded from experts, such as behavioural healthcare practitioners [54].

[55] present a list of difficulties in rural areas where telehealth can help in the following ways:

1. The discrepancy in the provision of health care between rural and urban areas is "mainly because of the difficulty of creating, maintaining and keeping adequately and properly trained rural health workers". Telehealth has the potential to narrow this gap by giving remote individuals access to additional healthcare services.
2. Healthcare policymakers who wish to improve rural population's access to care must find measures to increase the number and distribution of healthcare providers willing to work in remote areas.
3. Rural residents are often aged, sicker, and less sophisticated than city dwellers. Patients and professionals in rural areas can receive geriatric care and education through telehealth.
4. Despite considerable efforts by government and academic organizations to alleviate rural provider shortfalls over the last three decades, both the scarcity and misallocation of providers persist. Telehealth can help with distribution issues.
5. Health experts say "the more specialized you are, the more likely you are to settle in the city". Only family physicians are more likely to practise in rural communities that are smaller and more secluded. Telehealth has the potential to deliver specialist treatment to remote areas.

Telehealth has several advantages which includes [52], reduction in the cost of frequent doctor visits. It includes telecommunications, information technology and mobile technologies to provide healthcare services that allow patients and healthcare practitioners to consult across geographic boundaries. These might be innovations that are utilized by the users or physicians to improve or support telehealth services. Telehealth is being used in a variety of ways nowadays so that consultations between physicians and patients are made easier, [54] including transmission of data or images for analysis, remote monitoring, tele-pharmacy and enhanced provider communication. Obstruction of telehealth is as follows: [56,57]:

1. Healthcare practitioners must get a license where they plan to administer medications and visit patients.
2. In rural regions, there is a scarcity of high-speed data transfer capability.
3. Telecommunications administrations face substantial hardware and recurring expenditures.
4. Evidence-based barriers such as financial barriers – telehealth affordability to elderly individuals because of the cost of creating the infrastructure and lack of incentives to healthcare professionals.

M-health has risen because of the increased adoption and use of innovative, wireless and mobile technology to improve healthcare research, outcomes and services [58]. Table 8.2 shows a variety of m-health applications that are related to healthcare [59].

Voice over internet protocol (VOIP), internet access, voice calling, multimedia message service (MMS), text messaging and short message service (SMS) are all examples of m-health capabilities [60]. The most common m-health applications are sensors and point of care devices, client education and behaviour change, data collection and reporting, registries and vital event tracking, electronic decision-making assistance, electronic health records, communication between providers, work planning and scheduling for providers and provider education and training, management of the supply chain, human resource administration, and financial transactions and incentives [61]. m-health adoption is hampered by several obstacles.

TABLE 8.2
Healthcare Application Categories on m-Health

Categories	Applications
Depending on the on medical speciality	Family practice, forensic medicine, emergency medicine, immunology, allergy, infectious diseases, disability, pharmacology, internal medicine, palliative care, traumatology, intensive care, physical medicine and rehabilitation, public health, fitness.
Depending on area of studies	Doctoral associations, education, medical scientific literature, financial resources, biotech, emergency action systems, residential care organizations, policies governing public health, visualizing centres, GSM operators, hospitals, medical consultancy, association of patients, long-term assistance, data aggregation, health information system.
Depending on operation system	Android, iOS, BlackBerry, Windows.

The most significant stumbling block is the cost. Implementing such a technology-based system is expensive, and m-health systems can only become mainstream if the government and health insurance companies allocate cash for this investment. According to the WHO report, privacy and security are an additional challenge for m-health systems. Another hurdle is logistics, as some rural areas still lack internet connectivity due to logistical issues.

Electronic healthcare (e-healthcare) has grown as a radical new approach because of rapid developments in information and communication technologies [62]. E-healthcare is increasingly displacing traditional healthcare and promoting the creation of innovative healthcare applications because of technological advancements [63]. IoT is becoming increasingly important in the ever-changing healthcare landscape [64]. The Internet of Things (IoT) is a new paradigm that allows them to integrate and communicate with objects or objects such as RFID (Radio Frequency Identification) sensors, cell phones, tags and actuators. Devices and people connect, communicate, gather and share data through integrating physical things, hardware, software and computational devices in e-healthcare, which is designated as the Internet of Healthcare Things (IoHT) [65]. Connecting the digital and physical worlds [66], IoT uses ubiquitous and pervasive computing, as well as e-healthcare platforms, to enable healthcare devices (e.g. mobile devices, fitbits, Bluetooth, sensors, etc.) to accumulate health related data (e.g. glucose level, blood pressure, blood oxygen saturation, weight, respiratory and heart rate, and so on) [67, 68] over a long period and store it. There are several areas of healthcare where the IoT plays an important role [69].

- Elderly care including housing / patient monitoring of elderly people in nursing homes and hospitals.
- It includes several pieces of equipment which is seen at bedsides in hospitals, such as the monitoring of electrocardiogram, the data collection of which is the most matured field for healthcare and an area which continues to increase with new advancements in IoT.
- At a reduced cost, real-time location is used to track people and assets.

Hadoop clusters may be used to process healthcare data in the cloud. Applications running on scalable servers can accommodate a significant number of participants [70]. The result data can be transferred to the cloud and the data can be integrated by Hadoop MapReduce in many servers on the cloud and managed to produce the results rapidly as shown in Figure 8.6. Deep learning breakthroughs based on convolutional neural networks have empowered significant gains in a variety of activities such as identification of images [71], interpretation of speech [72], discovery of drugs [73] and cancer research using gene analysis [74, 75]. Table 8.3 shows some of the applications of healthcare domain, as well as their pros and cons.

Fog computing collects and processes massive quantities of raw data produced by IoT / end devices, allowing for real-time analysis and decision making in the present circumstances. End devices continue to collect data to monitor the environment. As a result, the fog nodes must import data from the end node in real time. In some applications, such as body area networks, body sensors would upload massive amounts of data on a regular basis. Data processing, such as data filtering, data

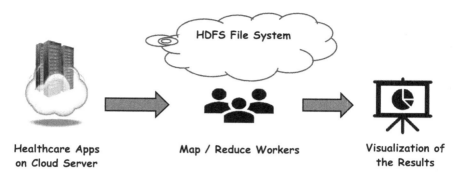

Healthcare Apps   Map / Reduce Workers   Visualization of
on Cloud Server   the Results

FIGURE 8.6   Healthcare data processing on a cloud server [70].

TABLE 8.3
Machine/Deep Learning Mechanisms Used in the Healthcare Domain

Algorithms Used	Healthcare Examples	Pros/Performance Metrics Used	Cons
Fully convolutional residual network [76]	Dermoscopic images	To classify melanoma, a very deep residual network of about 16 blocks is used, accuracy.	Multiscale contextual information integration, to integrate probabilistic graphical models in the network.
Deep learning [77]	Electronic health records	Predicting readmission for heart failure by finding critical factors. Precision, F-1 score, accuracy, recall.	Labelling of the admission as positive and negative
U – Net deep learning [78]	Electron and optical microscopy images	Segmentation on neuronal structures in EM stacks and cell tracking, very good segmentation performance even with limited data, Rand – error.	Data size is small of 30 images, training time of model is high.
C5.0 decision tree [79]	Pathological, demographic characteristics, physiological fertility, genetic and disease history and behavioural habits.	The cost matrix in the C5.0 model has been substantially improved. The performance metrics used are accuracy, specificity, sensitivity.	The dataset used is small, cancer is highly concealed and unclear, and the data set contains a large number of samples with minor illness features.

TABLE 8.3 (Continued)
Machine/Deep Learning Mechanisms Used in the Healthcare Domain

Algorithms Used	Healthcare Examples	Pros/Performance Metrics Used	Cons
Ensemble and transfer learning [80]	X-Ray Images	On two big datasets, cancer prediction was tested against human readers, AUC – ROC.	Use of simulation tool in AI
Two stage FCN [81]	MRI Images	Detects candidate microbleeds before to reduce false positives, can be easily applied to another biomarker detection task.	Excludes the phase information which includes the possible mimics of calcifications
CNN with fully connected CRF [82]	MRI Images	TBI, brain tumours, and ischemic stroke are all segmented on a multi-scale basis, Haussdorf, Precision, Sensitivity,	Dense inference on entire volume requires a forward-pass, Tiling the volume into multiple segments.

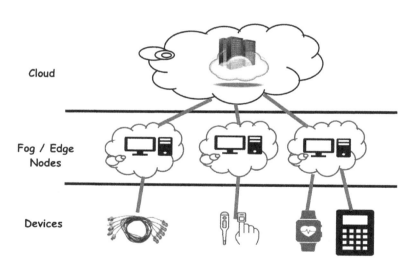

FIGURE 8.7   Fog computing architecture [83].

accumulation, and so on, needs to be performed by fog nodes. For instance, the ECG sensors will handle the emergency data quickly, in accordance with local policy, in the fog node. The steps are depicted in a straightforward manner in Figure 8.7 [83]. Since fog can provision on-site data storage, it can perform intelligent computations and investigation of these data, as well as disseminate some policy-based choices to the respective industry to promote better performance.

It is possible that if the end device is hooked up to the internet and generates data, it will not be essential to transmit or sync the information to the cloud due to redundant data [84]. The cloud keeps its primary "brain-trust" role in the fog model (evaluating information and making all of the major choices). The cloud, on the other hand, can delegate some duties to fog nodes, making it ideal for edge analysis and decision-making. Additionally, if the fog does not require in-depth analytics, they can simply sieve local data and preferentially send it to the cloud [85]. As a result, the transmission efficiency of widely spread sensor networks may be significantly improved.

8.6.2 Applications for Healthcare Professionals

These applications can assist healthcare professionals to improve their working environment, automate tedious chores and provide increasingly sophisticated services to help them do their jobs even better. Because healthcare applications collect, store and analyse massive quantities of data, they will also gather information on employees and how they execute their jobs. In a variety of ways, this information may be used to power programmes that optimize and improve people management.

1. **Scheduling**: several factors make scheduling professional healthcare staff, such as doctors, surgeons, nurses and therapists, extremely difficult to achieve an ideal timetable. In addition to the factors such as start and end time, location, and vacations, speciality, experience level, the condition of the patient, shifts, demand fluctuations and needed resource availability must all be into consideration. Healthcare applications can be intended to pull information about the faculty, assets, request levels and even chronicled information and utilize progressed algorithms to make enhanced timetables, make alternate courses of action and, furthermore, represent potential crises. This method will assist with giving the experts better timetables, more unsurprising prerequisites, and further developed workplace.

2. **Access to resources**: a lot of resources are needed to accomplish tasks by healthcare workers. Doctors and nurses, among many other resources, are most essential. They need counselling rooms, diagnostic devices, operation rooms and a variety of other resources. Certain approvals may be required for assigning and providing access to certain of these resources, or there may be a restricted amount of specific resources that may need scheduling.

3. **Alliance**: different areas of the medical system require collaboration between staff within the same organization, between facilities in the same organization, or with other systems and units. Based on the situation of the patient, doctors need to consult with one another on some cases and from different organization as well. Administrators need to share the information or work-related information to manage the overall working of the organization. The administrators

TABLE 8.4
Different Types of IoT Devices Used in Healthcare Applications

Healthcare Applications	Type of Sensor Used	Functioning of Sensor
Monitoring of patient [86]	Temperature sensor, respiration rate sensor, pulse rate sensor.	Sensors used in this application measure a person's body temperature, pulse rate and breath rate.
Stress detection [87]	ECG Monitoring sensors, accelerometer.	Collects the ECG signals and measures the angle between user and object.
Position altering [88]	Accelerometer, pulse sensor and ultrasonic sensor.	Used to measure the heart rate, angle between the objects and determines the tilt angle between the person and the entity.
Paralyzed [89]	Infrared sensor.	Acts as a comparator.
Visually challenged [90]	Ultrasonic sensor.	It is used to figure out how far apart two items are.
Home monitoring [91]	CO_2 sensor.	Measures CO_2 content levels.
Elderly monitoring [92]	Light sensor, airflow sensor, oximeter sensor.	Detects light, monitors the amount of oxygen in the blood and detects haemoglobin.
Military [93]	Sensor to detect the explosives.	Detects explosives.
Alcohol detection [94]	PID sensor.	Detects the chemical content.
Diabetes monitoring [95]	Weight and pressure sensors.	Detects the body weight.

also need to collaborate with the health equipment manufacturers, transportation companies, insurance companies, drug manufacturers, suppliers of consumables and healthcare services.

4. **Remote access**: Most of the organizations are small and cannot afford sophisticated and expensive equipment. Specialised facilities have their own expertise and equipment. Having a simple and secure means to access and utilise such equipment will be a huge assistance to the requester, allowing them to reap even more advantages from it. Some applications may be to request to use the radiology reports to analyse their results. Table 8.4 shows the different IoT devices such as sensors used in the healthcare system.

8.6.3 APPLICATIONS FOR RESOURCE MANAGEMENT

The healthcare systems as a whole is huge and contains thousands of assets. These include furniture and other fixtures, as well as physical infrastructure and related service units such as heating, ventilation, and Air Conditioning (HVAC) such as water, oxygen, electrical and fire alarm systems. Healthcare organizations also have components such as laboratory and diagnostic equipment, sanitizing material, medication treatment tools, security instruments and material, surgical materials and equipment, and food.

1. **Accessibility**: when resources are required, they must be available. Hospital beds, life support equipment, pharmaceuticals and even personnel will be in limited supply during emergencies such as terrorism, pandemic or natural disasters. And in some situations, resources may not be available due to expiry date, due to failures, maintenance, reallocation and misuse.
2. **Sharing**: in order to carry out the processes that need resources, particularly essential and shared resources must be assigned to their appropriate healthcare professionals. The organization shares operation theatres, MRI scanners, X-Ray machines and ICU equipment across various departments such as OPD, Cardiology, Anaesthesiology, Orthopaedics, Paediatrics, etc.
3. **Connectivity**: all the devices in the healthcare applications must be linked using some technologies such as wired, wireless, Bluetooth, NFC, etc. The provision of connectivity-based resources will make better use of them and details on the resources, their capacities, status and usage history more easily accessible.
4. **Maintenance of equipment**: maintenance management's specific goals of are as follows: [96] to boost the dependability of infrastructure and equipment, to keep equipment and infrastructure in good working order at all times, to make emergency repairs to equipment and infrastructure as soon as feasible in order to ensure the highest possible availability for medical usage, to enhance operational security, and to educate medical professionals on precise control techniques, to provide guidance on the purchase, installation and operation of medical devices and to provide medical insurance and environmental protection.

8.7 SECURITY AND PRIVACY

On the basis of data, communication, and device anonymity properties, the privacy goals are considered [97 – 99].

1. **Anonymity of the device**: the identification of medical equipment must be hidden to the system, such that unauthorised entities ought not to be able to identify the precise device identifier, device type, and conventional identifiers such as MAC address and IP address.
2. **Data cloaking**: the purpose of information anonymization is to stop intruders from being able to identify a user and their sensitive data. Medical professionals should use pseudonyms or another temporary identifier's rather than their actual identity.
3. **Anonymity of the communication**: an unauthorized entity cannot determine the connection between the end-user and the healthcare system. To ensure

anonymous communication, effective techniques such as collision-resistant aliases should be employed.

4. **Link ability**: an intruder who records information exchange between transmission and reception should not be in a position to establish a connection between the sender and the information.

8.8 CONCLUSION

Healthcare is a major problem for any country's or individual's overall economic and development progress. The analytics is deepening into the medical fabric and will shape the future of medicine and care delivery. Various types of data are needed in the healthcare system to allow seamless communication between the doctors and patients, to improve patient engagement in the treatment process, to offer evidence-based care, and to detect security risks and fraud early. The emergence of digital platforms such as mobile devices, cloud computing, analysis of data, and wireless networks have contributed to the effective delivery of medical services, analyse trends and disease, and make better policy decisions. The blockchain ledger allows the safe transfer of patient information, the management of the medication supply chain, and the assistance of healthcare researchers in solving the problems. In this chapter we have outlined the architecture of cloud and fog architectures of healthcare applications, various types of data, summarized the various applications in the healthcare industry, the use of blockchain technology in the healthcare domain, the research gap and challenges in cancer imaging, fall detection and research and clinical procedures. Once new solutions for research gaps and challenges are applied in clinical practice, healthcare informatics are expected to raise the quality of care levels, possibly revolutionising precision medicine.

REFERENCES

[1] M. Pavel, H. B. Jimison, H. d. Wactlar, T. L. Hayes, W. Barkis, J. Skapik, & J. Kaye, The role of technology and engineering models in transforming healthcare. IEEE Reviews in Biomedical Engineering, 6, 156–177, 2013.

[2] M. Tahar Kechadi, Healthcare big data: challenges and opportunities, BDAW'16, November 10–11, 2016, Blagoevgrad, Bulgaria, ACM.

[3] R. Nallusamy & R. Asija, A survey on security and privacy of healthcare data, 2015, Conference paper. doi:10.5176/2251-3833_GHC14.29.

[4] M. Asif-Ur-Rahman, F. Afsana, M. Mahmud, M. S. Kaiser, M. R. Ahmed, O. Kaiwartya, & A. James-Taylor, Towards a heterogeneous mist, fog, and cloud based framework for the Internet of Healthcare Things. IEEE Internet of Things Journal, 2018, 1–1.

[5] I. Olaronke & O. Oluwaseun, Big data in healthcare: Prospects, challenges and resolutions. Future Technologies Conference, 2016. doi:10.1109/ftc.2016.7821747.

[6] S. Jeong, C.-H. Youn, E. Bo Shim, M. Kim, Y. Min Cho, & L. Peng, An integrated healthcare system for personalized chronic disease care in home–hospital environments. IEEE Transactions on Information Technology in Biomedicine, 16(4), 2012, 572–585.

[7] C. Burghard, Big data and analytics key to accountable care success, IDC Health Insights, 2012.

[8] B. Qureshi, Towards a digital ecosystem for predictive healthcare analytics. Proceedings of the 6th International Conference on Management of Emergent Digital EcoSystems – MEDES, 2014. doi:10.1145/2668260.2668286.

[9] M. J. Kaur & V. P. Mishra, Analysis of big data cloud computing environment on healthcare organizations by implementing Hadoop clusters. 2018 Fifth HCT Information Technology Trends, 2018. doi:10.1109/ctit.2018.8649546.

[10] C. He, X. Fan, & Y. Li, Toward ubiquitous healthcare services with a novel efficient cloud platform. IEEE Transactions on Biomedical Engineering, 60(1), 230–234, 2013.

[11] Y. Liu, L. Zhang, Y. Yang, L. Zhou, L. Ren, F. Wang, R. Liu, Z. Pang, & M. Jamal Deen, A novel cloud-based framework for the elderly healthcare services using digital twin, 2019, Healthcare Information Technology for the Extreme and Remote Environments, IEEE Access, pp 49088–49101.

[12] C. O. Rolim, F. L. Koch, C. B. Westphall, J. Werner, A. Fracalossi, & G. S. Salvador, A cloud computing solution for patient's data collection in health care institutions. 2010 Second International Conference on eHealth, Telemedicine, and Social Medicine, 2010. doi:10.1109/etelemed.2010.19.

[13] Y. Shi, G. Ding, H. Wang, H. E. Roman, & S. Lu, The fog computing service for healthcare. 2015 2nd International Symposium on Future Information and Communication Technologies for Ubiquitous HealthCare (Ubi-HealthTech), 2015. doi:10.1109/ubi-healthtech.2015.7203325.

[14] E. Badidi & K. Moumane, Enhancing the processing of healthcare data streams using fog computing. 2019 IEEE Symposium on Computers and Communications, 2019. doi:10.1109/iscc47284.2019.896973.

[15] M. H. Kuo, T. Sahama, A. W. Kushniruk, E. M. Borycki, & D. K. Grunwell, Health big data analytics: current perspectives, challenges and potential solutions. International Journal of Big Data Intelligence, 1(1/2), 114, 2014.

[16] E. Xu, J. Mei, J. Li, Y. Yu, S. Huang, & Y. Qin, From EHR data to medication adherence assessment: a case study on Type 2 diabetes. IEEE International Conference on Healthcare Informatics, 2019. doi:10.1109/ichi.2019.8904786.

[17] C. I. Sheriff, T. Naqishbandi, & A. Geetha, Healthcare informatics and analytics framework, 2015 International Conference on Computer Communication and Informatics. doi:10.1109/iccci.2015.7218108.

[18] R. S. Evans, Electronic health records: then, now, and in the future, 2016, NCBI, PMC, US National Library of Medicine, National Institute of Health.

[19] V. Chandola, S. R. Sukumar, & J. C. Schryver, Knowledge discovery from massive healthcare claims data. Proceedings of the 19th ACM SIGKDD International Conference on Knowledge Discovery and Data Mining, 2013. doi:10.1145/2487575.2488205.

[20] G. J. Katuwal, S. Pandey, M. Hennessey, & B. Lamichhane, Applications of Blockchain in Healthcare: Current Landscape & Challenges, 2018.

[21] M. Nagori, A. Patil, S. Deshmukh, G. Vaidya, M. Rahangdale, C. Kulkarni, & V. Kshirsagar, Mutichain enabled EHR management system and predictive analytics, in Smart Trends in Computing and Communications. Singapore: Springer, 2020, pp. 179–187.

[22] E. Gökalp, M. Onuralp Gökalp, S. Çoban, & P. Erhan Eren, Analysing opportunities and challenges of integrated blockchain technologies in healthcare, 2018, 174–183, Springer Nature Switzerland AG.

[23] X. Wang, J. Ellul & G. Azzopardi, Elderly Fall Detection Systems: A Literature Survey, Frontiers, Robotics and AI (frontiersin.org)

[24] S. R. Islam, D. Kwak, M. H. Kabir, M. Hossain, & K.-S. Kwak, The internet of things for health care: a comprehensive survey. IEEE Access 3, 678–708, 2015.

[25] W. L. Bi et al., Artificial intelligence in cancer imaging: clinical challenges and applications, ACS, 69, 2, 2019.

[26] M. S. Ferdous, K. Biswas, M. J. M. Chowdhury, N. Chowdhury, & V. Muthukkumarasamy, Integrated platforms for blockchain enablement, Advanced Computing, no. March, 2019.

[27] U. Goel, R. Ruhl, & P. Zavarsky, Using healthcare authority and patient blockchains to develop a tamper-proof record tracking system, 2019 IEEE 5th Intl Conference on Big Data Security on Cloud (BigDataSecurity), IEEE Intl Conference on High Performance and Smart Computing (HPSC), and IEEE Intl Conference on Intelligent Data and Security (IDS).

[28] T. K. Dasaklis, F. Casino, & C. Patsakis, Blockchain meets smart health: towards next generation healthcare services. 2018 9th International Conference on Information, Intelligence, Systems and Applications, 2018. doi:10.1109/iisa.2018.8633601.

[29] M. Mettler, Blockchain technology in healthcare: the revolution starts here, 2016 IEEE 18th International Conference on e-Health Networking, Applications and Services, Healthcom 2016, pp. 16–18, 2016.

[30] A. Azaria, A. Ekblaw, T. Vieira, & A. Lippman, MedRec: using blockchain for medical data access and permission management, 2016 2nd International Conference on Open and Big Data (OBD), Vienna, pp. 25–30, 2016.

[31] C. D. Parameswari & V. Mandadi, Healthcare data protection based on blockchain using solidity, Fourth World Conference on Smart Trends in Systems, Security and Sustainability, 2020. doi:10.1109/worlds450073.2020.921.

[32] Waves whitepaper, 2018. https://blog:wavesplatform:com/waves-whitepaper-164dd 6ca6a23.

[33] D. Duffield, Dash: A payments-focused cryptocurrency, 2018. https://github:com/dashpay/dash/wiki/Whitepaper.

[34] The BitShares Blockchain, 2018. https://github:com/dashpay/dash/wiki/Whitepaper.

[35] A. Farouk, A. Alahmadi, S. Ghose, & A. Mashatan, Blockchain platform for industrial healthcare: vision and future opportunities, Computer Communications, 2020, Elsevier, pp 223–235.

[36] M. Pilkington, Blockchain technology: principles and applications, in: Research Handbook on Digital Transformations, Edward Elgar Publishing, 2016.

[37] Z. Zheng, S. Xie, H. Dai, X. Chen, & H. Wang, An overview of blockchain technology: Architecture, consensus, and future trends, in: 2017 IEEE International Congress on Big Data, Big Data Congress, IEEE, 2017, pp. 557–564.

[38] S. Nakamoto, Bitcoin: A Peer-to-Peer Electronic Cash System, 2019, Manubot.

[39] K. Salah, R. Jayaraman, & Y. Al-Hammadi, Blockchain for healthcare data management: opportunities, challenges, and future recommendations, 2021, Neural Computing and Applications. doi:10.1007/s00521-020-05519-w.

[40] D. Ichikawa, M. Kashiyama, & T. Ueno, Tamper-resistant mobile health using blockchain technology, JMIR mHealth uHealth, Vol 5 (7), 2017.

[41] K. N. Griggs, O. Ossipova, C. P. Kohlios, A. N. Baccarini, E. A. Howson, & T. Hayajneh, Healthcare blockchain system using smart contracts for secure automated remote patient monitoring, J. Med. Syst. 42 (7) (2018) 130.

[42] J. H. Tseng, Y. C. Liao, B. Chong, & S. W. Liao, Governance on the drug supply chain via gcoin blockchain, International Journal of Environmental Research and Public Health, Vol 15 (6), 2018.

[43] M. Benchoufi, R. Porcher, & P. Ravaud, Blockchain protocols in clinical trials: transparency and traceability of consent, F1000Research 6, 2017.

[44] Z. Shae & J. J. Tsai, On the design of a blockchain platform for clinical trial and precision medicine, in: 2017 IEEE 37th International Conference on Distributed Computing Systems, ICDCS, IEEE, 2017, pp. 1972–1980.

[45] HIMSS Clinical & business intelligence: an analytics executive review, 2013. http://himss.files.cmsplus.com/HIMSSorg/Content/files/HIMSS%20CBI%20 Analytics%20Exec%20 Review_Industry%20Capabilities%20module_2013-02-19_FINAL.pdf.

[46] P. Sulkers, Healthcare analytics: a game-changer for North York General Hospital. Canadian Healthcare Technology, 2011. www-03.ibm.com/industries/ca/en/healthcare/ documents/NYGH_article_reprint_Cdn_Healthcare_Technology_July%202011.pdf.

[47] C. I. Sheriff, T. Naqishbandi, & A. Geetha, Healthcare informatics and analytics framework. 2015 International Conference on Computer Communication and Informatics, 2015. doi:10.1109/iccci.2015.7218108.

[48] G. Chen & M. Islam, Big data analytics in healthcare. 2019 2nd International Conference on Safety Produce Informatization, 2019. doi:10.1109/iicspi48186. 2019.9095872

[49] I. K. Kim, Z. Pervez, A. M. Khattak, & S. Lee, Chord based identity management for e-healthcare cloud applications. 2010 10th IEEE/IPSJ International Symposium on Applications and the Internet, 2010. doi:10.1109/saint.2010.68.

[50] P.-Y. S. Hsueh, R. J. R. Lin, M. J. H. Hsiao, L. Zeng, S. Ramakrishnan, & H. Chang, Cloud-based platform for personalization in a wellness management ecosystem: why, what, and how. Proceedings of the 6th International ICST Conference on Collaborative Computing: Networking, Applications, Worksharing, 2010. doi:10.4108/icst.collaboratecom.

[51] J. Al-Jaroodi, N. Mohamed, & E. Abukhousa, Health 4.0: on the way to realizing the healthcare of the future, 2020, IEEE Access, 8, 2020, pp 211189–211210

[52] M. Bani Yassein, I. Hmeidi, M. Al-Harbi, L. Mrayan, & W. Mardini, IoT based healthcare systems: a survey, 2019, DATA '19: Proceedings of the Second International Conference on Data Science, E-Learning and Information Systems, December 2019, Article No.: 30, pp 1–9.

[53] S. S. Al-Majeed, I. S. Al-Mejibli, & J. Karam, Home telehealth by Internet of Things (IoT). 2015 IEEE 28th Canadian Conference on Electrical and Computer Engineering, 2015. doi:10.1109/ccece.2015.7129344.

[54] R. E. Gantenbein, Telehealth-based collaboration among primary and behavioral health care providers in rural areas, 2012 International Conference on Collaboration Technologies and Systems, 2012. doi:10.1109/cts.2012.6261094.

[55] E.H. Larson et al, State of the health workforce in rural america: profiles and comparisons. WWAMI Rural Health Research Center, University of Washington, Seattle, 2003.

[56] W. Mohamed & M. M. Abdellatif, Telemedicine: an IoT application for healthcare systems, ICSIE '19: Proceedings of the 2019 8th International Conference on Software and Information Engineering, April 2019, pp 173–177.

[57] S. Merkel & P. Enste, Barriers to the diffusion of telecare and telehealth in the EU: a literature review. IET International Conference on Technologies for Active and Assisted Living, 2015. doi:10.1049/ic.2015.0128.

[58] mHealth: new horizons for health through mobile technologies: second global survey on eHealth. Global observatory for eHealth series, 3. WHO Press, Geneva.

[59] G. Sariyer & M. Gokalp Ataman, Utilizing mHealth applications in emergency medical services of Turkey, 2018, Current and Emerging mHealth Technologies, Springer, Current and Emerging mHealth Technologies: Adoption, Implementation, and Use, Book Chapter.

[60] U. B. Nurmatov, S. H. Lee, B. I. Nwaru, M. Mukherjee, L. Grant, & C. Pagliari, The effectiveness of mHealth interventions for maternal, newborn and child health in low- and middle-income countries: protocol for a systematic review and meta-analysis. Journal of Global Health. 2014;4(1):010407

[61] A. Labrique, 12 common applications and a visual framework. Global Health: Science and Practice. 2013;1:1–12.

[62] A. Chehri, H. Mouftah, & G. Jeon, A smart network architecture for e-health applications, in Intelligent Interactive Multimedia Systems and Services. Berlin, Germany: Springer, 2010, pp. 157–166.

[63] S. F. Wamba, A. Anand, & L. Carter, A literature review of RFIDenabled healthcare applications and issues, Int. J. Inf. Manag., vol. 33, no. 5, pp. 875–891, 2013.

[64] S. M. R. Islam, D. Kwak, M. H. Kabir, M. Hossain, & K.-S. Kwak, The Internet of Things for health care: A comprehensive survey, IEEE Access, vol. 3, pp. 678–708, 2015.

[65] P. K. Verma et al., Machine-to-machine (M2M) communications: A survey, J. Netw. Comput. Appl., vol. 66, pp. 83–105, May 2016.

[66] P. Sethi & S. R. Sarangi, Internet of Things: architectures, protocols, and applications, J. Elect. Comput. Eng., vol. 2017, pp. 1–25, Jan. 2017.

[67] G. Acampora, D. J. Cook, P. Rashidi, & A. V. Vasilakos, A survey on ambient intelligence in healthcare, Proc. IEEE, vol. 101, no. 12, pp. 2470–2494, Dec. 2013.

[68] E. Spanakis et al., Connection between biomedical telemetry and telemedicine, in Handbook of Biomedical Telemetry. Hoboken, NJ, USA: Wiley, 2014, pp. 419–444.

[69] A. Chacko & T. Hayajneh, Security and privacy issues with IoT in healthcare, 2018, EAI Endorsed Transactions on Pervasive Health and Technology.

[70] M. J. Kaur & V. P. Mishra, Analysis of big data cloud computing environment on healthcare organizations by implementing Hadoop Clusters. 2018 Fifth HCT Information Technology Trends, 2018. doi:10.1109/ctit.2018.8649546.

[71] A. Elola, E. Aramendi, U. Irusta, A. Picón, E. Alonso, P. Owens, & A. Idris, Deep neural networks for ECG-based pulse detection during out-of-hospital cardiac arrest, Entropy 21 (3) (2019) 305.

[72] R. Miikkulainen, J. Liang, E. Meyerson, A. Rawal, D. Fink, O. Francon, B. Hodjat, et al., Evolving deep neural networks, in: Artificial Intelligence in the Age of Neural Networks and Brain Computing, Academic Press, 2019, pp. 293–312.

[73] N. Stephenson, E. Shane, J. Chase, J. Rowland, D. Ries, N. Justice, R. Cao, et al., Survey of machine learning techniques in drug discovery, Curr. Drug Metab. 20 (3) (2019) 185–193.

[74] K.K. Wong, R. Rostomily, & S.T. Wong, Prognostic gene discovery in glioblastoma patients using deep learning, Cancers 11 (1) (2019) 53.

[75] O. Klein, F. Kanter, H. Kulbe, P. Jank, C. Denkert, G. Nebrich, S. Darb-Esfahani, et al., MALDI-imaging for classification of epithelial ovarian cancer histotypes from a tissue microarray using machine learning methods, Proteom. Clin. Appl. 13 (1) (2019) 170018.

[76] L. Yu, H. Chen, J. Qin, & P.-A. Heng, Automated melanoma recognition in dermoscopy images via very deep residual networks, IEEE Trans. Med. Imag., vol. 36, no. 4, pp. 994–1004, Apr. 2017

[77] X. Liu, Y. Chen, J. Bae, H. Li, J. Johnston, & T. Sanger, Predicting heart failure readmission from clinical notes using deep learning. 2019 IEEE International Conference on Bioinformatics and Biomedicine, 2019. doi:10.1109/bibm47256. 2019.8983095.

[78] O. Ronneberger, P. Fischer, & T Brox, U-net: convolutional networks for biomedical image segmentation, in Proc. Medical Image Comput. Comp.-Assis. Interv. – MICCAI, Navab N., Hornegger J., Wells, W., & Frangi A. eds. Lecture Notes in Computer Science, vol. 9351, Cham: Springer, 2015

[79] Xia Zhang & Yingming Sun, Breast cancer risk prediction model based on C5.0 algorithm for postmenopausal women, 2018, International Conference on Security, Pattern Analysis, and Cybernetics (SPAC), IEEE, Jinana, China.

[80] S. M. McKinney et al., International evaluation of an AI system for breast cancer screening, Nature, vol. 577, pp. 89–94, 2020

[81] Q. Dou et al., Automatic detection of cerebral microbleeds from MR images via 3D convolutional neural networks, IEEE Transactions on Medical Imaging., vol. 35, no. 5, pp. 1182–1195, May 2016.

[82] K. Kamnitsas et al., Efficient multi-scale 3D CNN with fully connected CRF for accurate brain lesion segmentation, Med. Image Anal., vol. 36, pp. 61–78, 2017.

[83] Y. Shi, G. Ding, H. G. Wang, H. E. Roman, & S. Lu, The fog computing service for healthcare. 2015 2nd International Symposium on Future Information and Communication Technologies for Ubiquitous HealthCare, 2015. doi:10.1109/ ubi-healthtech.2015.7203325.

[84] M. Aazam, P. Hung, & E. Huh, Smart gateway based communication for cloud of things [C]. IEEE, 2014:1–6.

[85] Fog Computing—clearly the way forward for IoT. http://blog.opengear.com/fog-computing-clearly-the-way-forward-for-iot.

[86] S. Biswas & S. Misra, Designing of a prototype of e-health monitoring system, pp 267–272.

[87] J. G. P. Rodrigues et al., A mobile sensing approach to stress detection and memory activation for public bus drivers, vol 6, pp. 3294–3303, 2015.

[88] N. Nowshin, M. Rashid, & T. Akhtar, Infrared sensor controlled wheel chair for physically disabled people, pp. 847–855, 2019.

[89] D. M. B, A. Celesti, M. Fazio, & M. Villari, Human-computer interface based on IoT embedded systems for users with disabilities, pp. 376–383, 2015.

[90] V. Bhatnagar, R. Chandra, & V. Jain, IoT Based Alert System for Visually Impaired, vol. 1. Springer Singapore.

[91] R. Pitarma, IAQ evaluation using an IoT CO_2 monitoring system for enhanced living environment, pp. 1169–1177, 2018.

[92] A. Abdelgawad, K. Yelamarthi, & A. Khattab, IoT-Based Health Monitoring System for Active and Assisted Living, vol. 1, pp. 11–20, 2017.

[93] A. Gondalia, D. Dixit, S. Parashar, & V. Raghava, ScienceDirect IoT-based healthcare monitoring system for war soldiers using machine learning, Procedia Computer Science vol. 133, pp. 1005–1013, 2018.

[94] Y. Umasankar, A. H. Jalal, P. J. Gonzalez, M. Chowdhury, S. Bhansali, & U. States, pp. 353–358, 2016.

[95] M. Saravanan & R. Shubha, Non-invasive analytics based smart system for diabetes monitoring, vol. 1, pp. 88–98, 2018.

[96] S. Duffuaa, A. Al Ghamdi, & A. Amer, Quality function deployment in maintenance work planning process. In: 6th Saudi Conference. Vol. 4. Dhahran, Kingdom of Saudi Arabia: KFUPM; 2002. pp. 503–5012

[97] S. Avancha, A. Baxi, & D. Kotz, Privacy in mobile technology for personal healthcare, ACM Computing Surveys (CSUR), vol. 45, no. 1, p. 3, 2012.

[98] A. R. Shahid, L. Jeukeng, W. Zeng, N. Pissinou, S. Iyengar, S. Sahni, & M. Varela-Conover, Ppvc: privacy preserving voronoi cell for location-based services, in 2017 International Conference on Computing, Networking and Communications (ICNC). IEEE, 2017, pp. 351–355.

[99] B. Yüksel, A. Küpçü, & Ö. Özkasap, Research issues for privacy and security of electronic health services, Future Generation Computer Systems, vol. 68, pp. 1–13, 2017.

9 Internet of Things-Healthcare System Architectures to Enhance the Healthcare Industry

Anil Audumbar Pise and Sangiwe Moyo
FinalMile Consulting City of Johannesburg, South Africa

CONTENTS

DOI: 10.1201/9781003145035-9

9.1 INTRODUCTION

Artificial Intelligence (AI) and the Internet of Things (IoT) are tying physical items and devices together because they encourage physical objects and devices to visualize, listen and think. Through the exchange of information, physical objects/devices are able to "speak" to one another and convey their decisions to one another. Products that were previously unintelligent are becoming intelligent thanks to technologies, for example, the IoT, which connect previously unintelligent objects to the internet by using a variety of embedded devices, sensor networks, communication protocols, internet protocols and also applications to connect them to the internet. There are several types of AI-based IoT, i.e. AIoT-enabled healthcare services being used in the medical business, and they can be split into three categories: electronic health and telecare networks; diagnostic, preventive and other associated technologies; and other related technologies. There are also plans to install equipment for rehabilitation and monitoring purposes. Internet of Things components like a Wi-Fi body area network and radio frequency recognition systems, for example, contribute to the functioning of the system but are not essential to its operation as a whole. While researches in neighbouring fields has demonstrated that remote-health tracking is viable, the potential advantages in a range of situations are maybe even more significant to consider in light of the findings, which should be explored in greater depth. Remote health surveillances, when utilized to track non-critical patients based at home rather than in the hospitals, can help to minimize the demand on hospital resources, for example, physicians and beds, hence reducing the demand on hospital resources. It can be utilised, for example, to increase access to healthcare for remote communities or to allow aged peoples to live in their homes for longer periods of time. The prospect for increased access to healthcare services, while simultaneously reducing the pressure on healthcare institutions, is a positive development. This is paramount, given the global shortage of healthcare workers and emerging infectious diseases. Moreover, it has the potential to empower individuals by enabling them to keep greater control over their own well-being at any time, thereby moving populations to selfcare options which have the potential to make health services more sustainable with less reliance of government interventions in the care continuum. Figure 9.1 displays a graphical representation of Internet of Things-based healthcare equipment that is currently in use in the healthcare sector.

Presently, healthcare system depends on a patchwork of heterogeneous and continuous monitoring equipment which provide warnings in the case of major occurrences using single physiological waveform data or discretized essential data [2]. Such straightforward ways to building and deploying alarm systems, on the other hand, are intrinsically untrustworthy, and their absolute number may cause "alarm fatigue" in either caregivers and patients [3, 4]. In this situation, past information

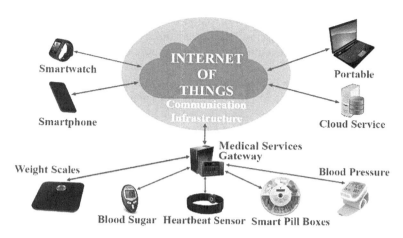

FIGURE 9.1 IoT-based healthcare devices [1].

which has frequently fallen short of properly leveraging high-dimensional time series data limits the possibility for new medical knowledge development. The reason these warning systems typically fail, according to Jerry et al., is that they depend on restricted sources of data and lacked a framework on the patients' genuine physiological circumstances from a larger and more complete lookout [5]. As an outcome, more comprehensive and better methods for evaluating interaction and correlation between multimodal clinical time series data are needed. That's also crucial since research repeatedly shows that humans cannot explain about variations impacting more than two signals [6, 7].

It is widely recognized that the IoT holds promise for alleviating pressure on healthcare systems, and it has been the subject of several current studies [1]. A significant percentage of this study is devoted to monitoring people who have been diagnosed with certain illnesses, for example, diabetes [8] or Parkinson's disease [9]. The conduct of more studies will help achieve several goals, including assisting in the rehabilitation of patients by continuously monitoring their development [10]. Emergency healthcare has also been mentioned in similar works [11], but has gained little publicity thus far.

A large amount of research has been conducted with a particular focus on recovery following physical injury. Reference [12] describes the development of a framework that results in the development of a recovery approach tailored to the symptoms of a specific individual. To accomplish this, the patient's diagnosis is linked to a record that contains information about previous patients' indicators, illnesses and cures, and it is important to mention genetic profiling as well. Manually inputting symptoms and authorizing prescribed medication is possible using this method; in 87.9 percent of cases, the doctor monitored the suggestions of the system completely and made no changes to the care plan it recommended. In [13], the value of current IoT technology is evaluated in context of a strategy for tracking Parkinson's disease patient. After conducting their research, the researchers came to the conclusion that wearable monitors proficient of detecting gait habits, tremble and common activity threshold might be practiced in conjunction with vision-based systems (i.e. cameras) installed in the home to identify the onset of Parkinson's disease. Moreover, the authors argue that machine learning may eventually give rise to more effective treatment strategies for cancer patients.

A practical method for diabetic patients to monitor their blood glucose levels was proposed by the author in [14]. Patients must manually obtain blood glucose measurements at predefined intervals under the conditions of this treatment. Following that, it goes into detail on two different types of blood glucose abnormalities. High blood glucose levels are the first sign, and a blood glucose value that is not taken is the second. Additionally, based on the severity of the indiscretion, the procedure defines who must be alerted: the patient, his/her parents and family contacts, or emergency healthcare providers, for example, doctors and nurse practitioners. While this strategy is feasible and has been demonstrated to be workable, it might be made even more effective by automating the measurement of blood glucose levels. Authors [15], demonstrated a gadget for forecasting cardiac problems that was built using off-the-shelf components and a bespoke antenna, as was suggested by the researchers. The data from an ECG sensor is processed by a microcontroller, which allows the cardiac rhythm to be determined. This information is then communicated to the user's device via Bluetooth, where it is additionally processed and displayed in a user's apps. The authors point out that emerging procedures for heart attack prediction would advance the accuracy of the technique, including respiration rate monitoring, that has been demonstrated to support in the diagnosis of cardiac events, could result in even greater advancements [16].

9.1.1 CONTRIBUTION TO AIoT HEALTHCARE

1. There is a dearth of research on comparable endeavors; no systematic analysis of AIoT achievements in healthcare has been conducted to date.
2. Conducting a comparison of the effects of AIoT initiatives to those in other healthcare businesses, as other organizations have done.
3. Along with enhancing previous research, this study conducts a detailed evaluation of various categories of definite components of medical IoT advances.
4. According to the investigation's purpose, this research content will be shared with stakeholders who are interested in such technical improvements.

Technology has permeated several parts of today's healthcare systems, but much more work needs to be done before the desired results can be achieved. Medical sensor, remote healthcare assistance and bright solution for diagnosis and monitoring have all been demonstrated in case studies, but such systems are now only available in a restricted number of privileged hospital settings, according to the National Institutes of Health. The bulk of these solutions are also independent, and standalone solutions fall short of a centralized strategy, which is another issue to consider. Furthermore, most systems do not include benchmarking, which makes integration more challenging.

The remainder of this chapter has been structured as follows. Section 9.2 begins with a brief overview of AIoT in healthcare, followed by a problem statement. Section 9.3 delves into the Internet of Things (AIoT) and the interconnectedness of the healthcare sector. Section 9.4 summarizes the objectives and significant concerns in AIoT healthcare. Section 9.5 discusses AIoT goods, including smart stethoscopes, pacemakers, and defibrillators. Section 9.6 summarizes the analyses conducted for this study. This section examines how artificial intelligence is being utilized to enhance the delivery of humanitarian assistance during times of distress. The conclusion and future work are discussed in the following parts.

9.2 PROBLEM STATEMENT

The majority of recent writing on AIoT in healthcare has been on the technology's numerous applications in a variety of healthcare contexts, comprising nursing, ambient assisted living (AAL) and surgeries. Additionally, no trials have been conducted which studied AIoT advancements specifically in healthcare and then compare the findings to other healthcare sectors. As a continuation of a previous study, this article gives an exhaustive examination of the various classes of definite parts of AIoT developments in medicine, including the goal of presenting this knowledge to stakeholders with an interest in these types of advancements.

9.3 AIOT AND HEALTHCARE SYSTEM INTERCONNECTION

In the past patients communicated with healthcare providers: in person, over the phone, by text messaging or teleconferences. Patients were not receiving the most suitable medications due to the lack of a regular patient health evaluation routine for doctors and hospitals. Advanced technologies, which assist patient and doctor in maintaining their care and providing better care through the utilization of smart-devices enabled via the IoT, present novel opportunities for monitoring persons in the medical profession [17]. Patient participation and satisfaction have increased as a result of more transparent physician-patient contact. Moreover, the health of the patient might be tracked, which reduces the length of their hospital visit as well as risk of them returning to the hospital once they are discharged. The extensive utilisation of the IoT has the ability to diminish healthcare expenses and increase treatment effectiveness. In [18] Alves et al., also introduce statistical methods for assessing joint angles in physical hydrotherapy situations, allowing for the tracking of joint activity development over the period to be conducted. It is almost inevitable that the healthcare business will be revolutionized as a result of the IoT's capability to unite technology and people's actual bodies. This supports the healthcare sector as a whole because it benefits patients, family members, professionals and hospitals, among other things.

The healthcare industry is going through a tough situation right now. The growing senior population, the growth in chronic diseases, the rise in mental-disorders and the emergence of novel diseases are all having an impact on the whole excellence of healthcare facilities around the globe. The recent incident of the COVID-19 outbreak has had a significant impact on healthcare institutions and organizations around the world, emphasizing the incapacity of conventional ways to deal with similar dangers in the future in a timely manner [19]. The IoT and cloud services can assist the crumbling healthcare system during this time of need. However, during the work on establishing healthcare resolutions according to the Internet of Things and cloud services which has been happening for years, the necessity for fast prototyping and growth is becoming increasingly apparent as the world's perspective of healthcare threats shifts.

There have been several deep belief networks (DBNs) applied to sensor research on triboelectric sensors, including the research reported here, to draw out characteristics through the rare electrical impulses of a triboelectric keyboard and to conduct dynamic keystroke recognition [20]. However, in the absence of more artificial intelligence research, the results of the gait recognition experiment with a triboelectric sensor are regarded as preliminary at this time. To automatically classify gait types according to data acquired from gait pattern measurements, several approaches have been developed. According to numerous research studies these include, a one-dimensional (1D) convolutional neural network (CNN)-based technique which is particularly effective at extracting useful characteristics from smaller (fixed length) segments of a complete dataset, particularly when the position of the feature within the segment is unimportant. As a result, this method is particularly well suited for the analysis of temporal sequences of sensor data that have been divided into two categories as a result of this distinction: noisy states and stable states.

9.3.1 AIoT FOR HEALTH INSURANCE COMPANIES

Healthcare devices are becoming increasingly interconnected, necessitating the development of a variety of techniques to cope with the numerous scenarios that may happen as a result. Is it possible for insurance firms to use data from a health-monitoring device to assist with underwriting and operational chores, such as, is it probable for insurance companies to influence that information? They will be able to better identify and analyze prospective patient' accusations of fraud if they have this information, and they will be able to identify people who would benefit from this sort of treatment. An additional substantial benefit for clients is provided by insurance information technologies (IIT). Not only are they employed for the introduction of standard underwriting and pricing, they are also employed for the risk assessment [21]. Customers will be able to see the information that was used in each decision as a result of improved visibility, which will encourage decisions which are driven from the data. This enables organizations to perform in-based thinking in facets of their operations, increasing the understanding of their consumers of the reasoning behind each action. Figure 9.2 depicts a high-level overview of a typical Internet of Things-based healthcare system.

Incentives for exploiting and giving to the health data generated by IoT devices are being investigated by a large number of insurance companies. There are a variety of potential techniques for improving treatment compliance and more significantly increasing compliance among clients who use Internet of Things devices. They might give these facilities in interchange for their recorded action, which is something they

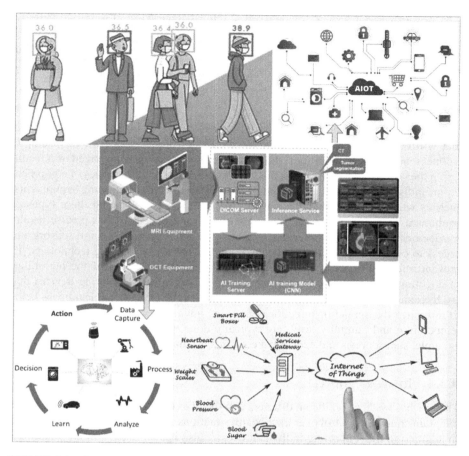

FIGURE 9.2   Overview of a typical AIoT-based healthcare system.

have complete control over, in exchange for their measured activity. This will also benefit insurance firms, who will be able to lower their liability claims as a result of this. These devices, similar to those which gather data from the IoT, might as well manage claims for insurance companies; it is possible that they will be able to show payment claims due to the insurance companies' participation.

9.3.2   IoT FOR PHYSICIANS

Wearable health-measuring and health-monitoring devices are utilised in conjunction with one another for extra precise recording of the health of the patient rather than separately. When using commercially accessible recordable clinical interventions, it is possible to determine whether or not a patient is fulfilling their medication objectives also while they are receiving treatment. Because of the Internet of Things, healthcare personnel may have a broader range of responsibilities in healthcare delivery, which may result in novel designs of interaction with patient. The information gathered by the gadgets supports healthcare practitioners in generating recommendations for their patients and gets to results which may be able to be predicted in advance of the procedure.

9.3.3 IoT for Hospitals

IoT will assist many people at healthcare facilities, but there are a slew of other things that will be more thoroughly monitored as a result of IoT adoption, for example, wellness and medical conditions, that might be more efficiently managed as a result. Using the sensor modules, it is possible to monitor and track these types of equipment on an individual basis. It is one instrument or remotely-transitioning equipments, such as wheelchair and nebulizer, which are beneficial for locating these types of equipment on a one-time basis. It is possible to obtain speedy and precise results for doctors and patients who are located at different locations thanks to sensors and access to cutting-edge equipment technology such as x-ray imaging technology. To prevent infection transmission, patients must be made conscious of the possibility of infection spread since it is important. The use of patient monitoring devices that are hygienic (safe) or that are related with hygienic (prophylactic) cleanliness helps to minimize the spread of infection. Assessing environmental factors, such as high temperature and humidity level, are typically done with the use of asset items, for example, smartphones and ecological control systems.

9.3.4 IoT for Patients

The IoT has made a significant difference in the lives of the elderly, allowing them to maintain complete control over their health situations 24 hours/day, seven days/week. In addition to this impacting individual lives, it also has an impact on their families, especially those who are single. If a patient gets released from the hospital and returns home, a notification is sent to respective family and any other medical practitioners who may need to know where the patient is so that they can be found and hospitalized if they require further treatment. Patients can monitor their state and keep track of their individual health better by using fitness bands and another wirelessly linked equipment, for example, blood pressure cuffs, blood pressure monitors and glucose sensors, which can be accessed by applications installed in their mobiles or another phones. Intended to calculate calories, record physical activity, take your blood pressure and achieve a variety of additional duties, these devices have the capability of remembering virtually everything.

9.4 OBJECTIVES AND KEY ISSUES IN IOT HEALTHCARE

The IoT is capable of bringing about significant advancements in healthcare as a result of its integration into healthcare programs. Furthermore, it is critical to begin thinking about the differences between the current structure and the environment of the future as early as possible. The two most crucial things to remember in this regard are to plan for the transition and to devote all of one's efforts to assisting the method in realizing its full potential. The necessity for interoperability is the first thing that springs to mind when thinking about this. In order to connect all agents and computers into a single huge network, uniform specifications and protocols must be developed. If higher-level standards and formats can be followed with greater quality in the future, it is in everyone's best interests to make concessions on them now while still allowing for future improvement. In order to manage such a massive volume of data, new standards must be established. The standardization of data forms and the use of networking technology are required to manage the huge amounts of data. The primary source of concern is that the "IoT" islands are kept apart from one another, which is a significant hurdle to them all combining into a single large "IoT".

While achieving the goal of having complete and comprehensive information may seem like an insurmountable challenge, one of the most significant roadblocks may be the implementation of a significant shift to an interconnected network in which information from the past is integrated into the current system. There are a variety of factors that contribute to the difficulty of data management in the medical industry. Furthermore, patient data is complex and/or deficient in specific areas, as previously stated. In addition, it supports a huge number of various storage formats, and its files are frequently kept in a variety of geographically separated locations. It is critical that we collect and organize healthcare data into useable repositories, establish databases that are consistent with existing standards, and make this data accessible to decentralized devices, enabling them to display and update it in real time or near real time. When dealing with this situation, paying close attention to the IoT is especially important because it may prove beneficial in assisting with the previously mentioned second goal.

The aims for this round are a function of the overall goal, which is to create healthcare that is more efficient, more successful, and more accessible to a broader section of the populace. Despite the fact that the structure for such an intervention already exists, the problem is determining how to continue in order to achieve the ultimate goal of delivering healthcare facilities that make the most of technological capabilities. When you think of change management, the theory that underpins it immediately comes to mind. According to the case study, this idea applies to businesses as well. For example, the move to a system that relies on interconnected data and devices to enable the flow of healthcare data among all providers demonstrates this [22].

9.5 AIOT HEALTHCARE DEVICES

Healthcare efforts that make use of IoT are in the works. The impact of limited healthcare resources on the lab technician workforce, as well as the reduction in the number of healthcare professionals as an outcome of deployment of health-related IoT devices, has the potential to ease the burden of the blood unavailability. Invasive, transdermal drugs, pacer systems, electronic gauge and another types of drug observers, in addition to supporting therapies, provide the capacity to assist doctors in diagnosing infections and tracking patient well-being. However, there are numerous advantages to expanding as well as numerous risks associated with doing so. Many people have brought up the topic of healthcare protection, which is something that everyone understands. It is possible for data thieves to access and steal information gathered and saved by embedded devices in the Internet of Things. Before widespread acceptance of Internet of Healthcare equipment and networks can be achieved, further expansion of the use of such equipment and networks is required. The applications of the IoT in universal healthcare are hampered by concerns about cybersecurity.

9.5.1 BLOOD COAGULATION TESTING

Roche invented a coagulation device that can communicate through Bluetooth. Patients might monitor the rate at which their blood clots using the Internet of Things technology. Roche's machine is the earliest Internet of Things machine that has been designed exclusively for patients who are anticoagulated. This strategy has been demonstrated to assist patients in maintaining inside their curing range while also decreasing their probability of bleeding and strokes. As a result of the ability to wirelessly send test information to their healthcare expert, patients saw their doctor less frequently. Additionally, Roche's device allows patients to annotate their test findings, tell them again to retest and alerts on test outcomes that fall outside of a predetermined range, among other features.

9.5.2 CONNECTED INHALERS

Asthma is a significant medical illness which affect lots of people all over world. People with asthma who use linked inhalers can raise their reservoir, providing them more control over their symptoms and treatment as they have state-of-the-art asthma-software. Propeller has developed a sensor which is able to control an inhaler or spirometer from a distance. Sensor is set up to notify patient with asthma and COPD about their thoughts and also facts that may aid them in making choices about their health. Sensor and software are used to notice medicine use and allergen presence, also to predict and alert customers about these changes. Some considered the attached inhaler as having significant benefits because it needs more effort on the part of the patient to utilize. The sensor also produces a report that can be referred to doctor's patient.

9.5.3 GLUCOSE MONITORING

For the more than 30 million diabetic Americans, glucose control has always been a concern. It takes time to manually monitor and document glucose levels, and it only notes a patient's glucose levels during the test. If levels change dramatically, routine monitoring is insufficient to detect a difficulty. IoT solutions that allow incessant, automated glucose monitoring of patients may help to relieve these concerns. Patients are notified when their blood glucose levels are irregular by glucose monitoring devices, which reduce the need for manual record keeping. Wireless implantable devices based on AIoT are depicted in Figure 9.3. Developing an AIoT system for glucose monitoring is one of the problems.

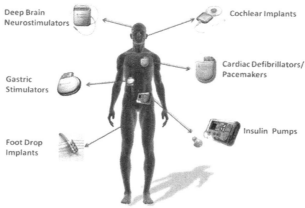

FIGURE 9.3   Wireless implantable medical devices [1].

One of the challenges is developing an AIoT system for glucose monitoring that:

1. The device is small enough to be used unobtrusively to track patients' progress over time without causing any inconvenience to the patients.
2. It doesn't consume so much energy that it needs to be invigorated on a consistent basis.

These are not insuperable problems, and devices that resolve them could change how people with diabetes control their blood sugar levels.

9.5.4   BLUETOOTH-ENABLED BLOOD LABS

The Swiss federal institute of technology, Lausanne, has developed implantable labs that allow for independent examination of patients' blood samples, giving crucial information. The implant is made up of five electrodes, each of which has an enzyme coating and can detect substances like glucose and lactate. The item is scanned and Bluetooth activated on the individual's PC when it is discovered. More research may be necessary. However, using a mobile connection, the results of this inquiry might be sent to a doctor in another place for evaluation. By reducing reliance on physicians, this big discovery would mostly assist the elderly and chronically ill. An implantable device removes the necessity for additional blood tests once it has been implanted, resulting in a decrease of lab personnel. An automated lab that removes the need for face-to-face interaction with patients reduces time spent gathering all essential lab tests, which helps the already overburdened healthcare system in a number of ways.

9.5.5   CONNECTED CANCER TREATMENT

The findings of a clinical study including patients with head and neck cancer were presented at the 2018 American Society of Clinical Oncology (ASCO) annual meeting in Chicago. In this pilot study, patients were wearing a Bluetooth device while receiving care, and their discomfort, heart rate and also weight were collected via Bluetooth and constantly monitored using a data collection software on blood pressure and pulse-tracking program, and the weight of each patient was counted every day to provide vital information to their physician. The drug may be modified on a daily basis if the doctor deems it necessary. Participants in the trial showed diminished symptoms when related to those in the placebo group who had never received any medical facilities related to cancer or individuals receiving medical facilities one time in a week.

Technology has aided in the simplification of patients' treatment by supporting with any developing side effects, and also labeling and alleviating their apprehensions, as well as enabling the recognition of effects caused by the implementation of advanced healthcare practices and the implementation of smart health practices. Smart technology therapies may lessen patients' issues and annoyance. It was found that more contact between patients and doctors makes healthcare better and cuts down on the time people spend in doctors' offices. This means that more people can do more everyday things.

9.5.6 ROBOTIC SURGERY

Through the use of tiny Internet-connected robots implanted into the human body, surgeons can do complex operations that would be hard to complete with human hands. At the same time, robotic surgeries performed by small Internet of Things devices would drastically minimize the size of incisions required for surgery, this will make the treatment less unpleasant and allow patients to recover more quickly.

9.5.7 IoT-CONNECTED CONTACT LENSES

A cataractophthins eye condition known as acquired longneess is likely to be cured using lens enlargement and lens stiffening treatments such as extra-capsular catarization in the future, according to current expectations. In order to treat long lens failure, also called presbyopia, which is responsible for long-flectomizedness, a research study will investigate lens healing or stiffening and refracting to make sure a recovery. Sensimed is a non-invasive device created by Swiss researchers that monitors changes in the pressures in the eyes that may indicate the onset of glaucoma. The signals are generated by a non-invasive device called Sensimed.

9.5.8 A SMARTWATCH APP THAT MONITORS DEPRESSION

Patients can utilize a tracking system on a regular basis to assess their emotions of depression, and one of the conditions for MDD is to wear a smartwatch on a daily basis. When looking at this scenario, there is an undeniably higher chance for wearable technologies to have a stronger impact on more than just step counting; gadgets that assess the intensity of depression will be acceptable in this situation. A depression app, like other Internet of Things applications, may assist patients and caregivers to gain additional information about their disorders.

9.5.9 CONNECTED WEARABLES

Without linked wearables, the Internet of Things looks to be incomplete. Since worn and linked sensors are important instruments for medical staff, it helps as well as assist patients. The use of such devices allows health personnel to monitor vital body statistics, for example, the heart rates, body temperature, pulses and other vital body data though still performing their duties and observing how individuals are doing. Aside from that, hospitals have the advantage of using wearable gadgets that maintain continuous contact with the wearer, allowing physicians to keep track of patients even after they have left the facility. In particular, it is useful in assisting patients with regular check-up appointments if they disclose concerns that they had while in the hospital after their discharge. If a condition varies, the wearable sensors will send an alert to the doctors, who will be able to respond from anywhere. Patients receive real-time guidance from their doctors when a real-time alert is issued to them by the medical system.

9.6 SUMMARY OF ASSOCIATED RESEARCH

Intelligent health-protection systems are a vital component of the development of intelligent cities. Promotional actions are being conducted to encourage the creation of a "digital health" system. Medical health big data platforms will be developed in the smart city to facilitate data distribution and exchange between medical and health service providers. A citizen medical health big-data centre will be developed on the smart city cloud platform to support three-medicine linkage as well as graded diagnosis and treatment. Furthermore, citizens of the city will have access to electronic health records, which will allow for the networking of medical services supplied by hospitals and clinics around the city to be implemented. Encourage the use of online registration, electronic toll collection, online telemedicine facilities, visual and physical examination diagnostic technologies, and other efforts targeted at improving the city's medical and health services to the greatest extent possible.

The current study looked into a number of different aspects of the IoT technology. It is the goal of this article to provide a comprehensive assessment of the AIoT system's architecture, components, and communication between these components. As an added bonus, this article describes existing healthcare services for which Internet of Things-based solutions have been investigated. Through the use of these ideas, IoT technology has assisted healthcare experts in monitoring and diagnosing a wide range of medical problems, evaluating a wide range of health indicators, and delivering diagnostic services in remote locations. A shift in emphasis away from hospital-centered methods and toward patient-centered strategies has resulted as a consequence of this transition. In addition, we discussed the many applications and current advances of artificial intelligence (AI) technology. Additionally, obstacles and concerns connected with the model, manufacturing and utilisation of the AIoT systems have all been solved. These tasks will serve as the foundation for the development and research objectives that will be pursued over the next several years. Additional extensive and up-to-date material on AIoT devices has been given for readers who want to not only begin their research but also expand their knowledge in the area has been included.

A fundamental reason for the quick development in relevance of the Internet of Things is the enormous benefits it provides in terms of higher precision, lower expenses, and the capability to predict upcoming events. Regardless of the fact that mobile phones and, for a long period, computer technology has been in use, the widespread accessibility of applications and the Internet of Things, as well as wireless technology and the virtual economy, have all contributed to the AIoT's speedy expansion, resulting in society's overall technology ecosystem continuing to enlarge [22].

In addition to AIoT products (which could be equipped with sensors, actuators, and so on), additional physical instruments (actuators, sensors, etc.) have been integrated in order to gather and communicate knowledge using protocols, for example, Bluetooth, Wi-Fi and IEEE 802.11 to do this [23]. Embedded or wearable sensors are also used in heart-related apps to collect clinical information about the patients. Examples of such sensors include a thermistor, a palpatory (a pressure sensor), an electrocardiogram (ECG) and an electroencephalogram (EEG), which measures the electric potential of the brain. Other environmental characteristics, such as temperature, humidity, date, time and day of the week, may also be recorded in addition to the above. These medical data may be utilised to generate intriguing and particular inferences about the clinical status of the patients based on their medical history. Considering that IoT sensors generate/capture many types of data from the internet, and that huge quantities of information are delivered by numerous sources, the AIoT is becoming increasingly important (sensors, e-mails, software, mobile phone and apps). The information acquired by the previous research is distributed to physicians, care takers and those who have been given permission to use the instruments. When the cloud or server style diagnosis and dispersion of these details with healthcare services is enlarged, it is a more effective use of the information, and treatments are provided more rapidly if they are needed.

At the moment, available options focus on sensors and smart refrigerators, both of which are still relatively new technologies. Temperature monitoring has long been required by safety regulations governing storage facilities. Monitoring the temperature of a refrigerator is not a novel notion, and with today's technological advancements and Internet of Things solutions, refrigerator temperature data may be monitored, stored in the cloud and evaluated.

Collaborative efforts are taking place between app users as well as between the healthcare organization and the contact module, which means that all parties have access to the app's data. It is human-interface-based that the majority of AIoT components (AIoT in the framework primarily serves as a dashboard for medical physicians and includes patients monitoring, data visualization and apprehension abilities) are implemented. By looking deeper into these challenges, the study indicated that AIoT in healthcare has improved on the findings from the previous year's study. Healthcare surveillance, government regulation, and privacy are three potential AIoT applications, and it would be good to begin by performing research into each of these areas first. These technological breakthroughs suggest that the IoT has the potential to be both productive and profitable in the healthcare industry. Maintaining quality-of-service conditions which enhance information exchange, steadiness, affordability and pliability though simultaneously safeguarding the privacy of all user information is, however, a difficult task to solve [24].

In Table 9.1, we looked at the contributions made by several research academics to the field of artificial intelligence in healthcare. The year 2019 saw the establishment of a cloud-based technique for conducting an AIoT analysis in healthcare by Dang et al. [18]. They made the decision to address many of the issues and concerns related to security, as well as the use of artificial intelligence and cloud computing in healthcare. In the year 2019, a significant number of peer-reviewed journal paper reviews were published [26], [26], [29], [30], [28] and 2018 [27], [25], both of which looked for publications prior to 2017. Nazir et al., conducted a comprehensive study of studies published between 2011 and 2019 that discussed the protection and privacy concerns of mobile-based healthcare IoT [28]. In the current state of affairs, there are no research studies dedicated explicitly to the use of medical artificial intelligence; nonetheless, relevant research papers on healthcare artificial intelligence are listed in Table 9.1. This table summarizes the findings of ten independent studies (including systemic analyses and other types of evaluations) that looked into the use of artificial intelligence in healthcare (AIoT) in more detail. The first study [21], researchers conducted a comprehensive AIoT review of healthcare, in which they looked at a variety of aspects of healthcare AIoT, including networks and architectures, procedures and implementations. Protection and standardization, as well as the Internet of Things and ehealth regulations and policies, were among the issues covered. Nevertheless, the information contained in this paper was written at a time when artificial intelligence was just getting started, and the need for it in the healthcare industry is expanding, prompting the construction of a new review.

A systematic [27] overview of the materials and innovations used in healthcare AIoT implementations was published in 2018 and we have shown in Table 9.1. As per the study, the home is the most prevalent location for healthcare AIoT. It reveals that Procedia Computer Science, the Journal of Network and Computer Applications, and the Journal of Medical Systems are the top-ranked journals for articles produced on the topic. Another research [31] from 2017 found that the hospital has been the most vulnerable location for AIoT acceptance. Certain countries' ehealth programs and strategies have been described as contributing to AIoT without providing readers with a summary of the countries' recognition contributions [21], [26]. Another issue that AIoT raises is security and confidentiality, as well as interoperability and integration with technology concerns in healthcare. We have discussed these topics in greater depth in previous papers [20], [21], [22], [25], [29], [32], [28], [33], and [34]. A variety of topics associated to the IoT in healthcare have been discussed in previous scholarly publications, including the application of numerous breakthroughs, for example, cloud computing, mobile computing, wearable sensors, fog computing and big data in the field, as well as the application of numerous breakthroughs such as big data in the field. Numerous research articles on the present status and possible advances in healthcare AIoT assess the existing situation as well as the potential for future advancements in healthcare.

TABLE 9.1
General Review of IoT in Healthcare

Paper Title	Contributions	Author and Year
The IoT for healthcare: a comprehensive survey	• Discussion of the issues and concerns linked with the IoT in the healthcare industry. • Incorporate IoT-related laws and regulations into your business strategy. Big data, ambient knowledge, and wearables are all topics to discuss in the healthcare industry. • Examine the network topologies and accompanying software or services in the IoT for healthcare applications.	Mahmud et al., [21] 2015
Medical Internet of Things and big data in healthcare	• Inspect the utilisation of IoT and big data in healthcare. • Deliberate the issues connected with the use of big data in healthcare. • Applications and mobile-phone applications for examination.	Dimiter [22] 2016
Internet of Things for smart healthcare: Technologies, challenges, and opportunities	• A description for the practice of IoT in healthcare is suggested. • The present state of affairs and likely upcoming developments in healthcare IoT are addressed. • Deliberate potential researches trends, issues, and problems of healthcare's IoTs. • Consider cloud computing as a data-storage system. • Pay attention to various wearable and networking devices.	Ian et al., [23] 2017
Advanced Internet of Things for personalised healthcare system: A survey	• Examine and categorize healthcare IoT systems, implementations, and positive case studies. • Give a four-layer IoT architecture for customized healthcare networks (PHS). • Deliberate future research developments, also concerns and difficulties in healthcare IoT. • Deliver a summary of the present situation and potential growths of healthcare IoT.	Xu et al., [24] 2017
Towards fog-driven IoT ehealth: Promises and challenges of IoT in medicine and healthcare	• Define a multi-tiered architecture for the IoT-enabled e-health ecosystem: To motivate, utilise devices, fog computing, and cloud-based services. • Deliberate how the IoT will be seen in hospitals and pharmacy. • Showcase a platform for the IoT-unified enabled ehealth world.	Nicholas et al., [25] 2018

TABLE 9.1 (Continued)
General Review of IoT in Healthcare

Paper Title	Contributions	Author and Year
A survey on Internet of Things and cloud computing for healthcare	• Conduct a research of the IoT structure for the healthcare sectors, with an importance on architecture, platform, and topologies. • Inspect the impact of IoT and cloud computing on healthcare. • Identify emerging market trends and initiatives in the realm of IoT and cloud computing in the healthcare business throughout the world. • Consider the security implications of IoT and cloud computing in healthcare.. • Study how the utilisation of IoT and cloud computing in healthcare poses a numbers of challenges.	**Min et al., [26] 2019**
The application of Inter-net of Things in healthcare: a systematicliterature review and classification	• Inspect the cybersecurity and interoperability concerns involved with healthcare IoT. • Express the present state of healthcare IoT and then current likely upcoming variations. • More about the IoT and how it could be included in healthcare. • Inspect the benefits of cloud-based architecture for IoT in healthcare.	**Reza et al., [27] 2019**
Internet of Things for healthcare using effects of mobile computing: a systematicliterature review	• Display the present state of healthcare IoT and then present possible upcoming variation. • Inspect the security and privacy issues posed by healthcare IoT. • Smartphone computing in healthcare IoT.	**Yasir et al., [28] 2019**
IoT-based healthcare applications: a review	• Express the present state of healthcare IoT and then current likely future changes. • Inspect the security and privacy issues posed by healthcare IoT. • Mobile computing in healthcare IoT.	**Gibeon et al., [29] 2019**
Enabling technologies for fog computing in healthcare IoT systems	• The present state of affairs and probable upcoming developments in healthcare IoT are addressed. • Gather either of their functioning and non-functional necessities. • Deliberate the concerns and queries around IoT structure in healthcare.	**Othman et al., [30] 2019**

9.7 APPLICATIONS OF IOT TO BUILD EMERGENCY MEDICAL SERVICES

Scholars also give to the growth of a reference model for IoT applications. A framework for organizing such a project is included in a research paper titled "Creating an IoT Implementation for Smart Cities" by Jin et al. [35], which was published in 2014. As stated in the article, the IoT will contribute to the creation of a smart city in three ways: datacentric IoT, cloud-centric IoT and network-centric IoT. The fact that they cover many of the different uses of smart development projects leads to their use as a reference model for creating smart cities as a result of their inclusion in this study. Figure 9.4 depicts a number of crucial areas of AIoT analytics in medicine that are highlighted.

9.7.1 DATA-CENTRIC IoT

This way of thinking focuses on data because there would be an enormous quantity of data produced by IoT gadgets if a big number of them were to be collected. With the term "Data-centric IoT," we mean that it describes the concept of all parts of the data flow, which includes the analysis of the information as well as the transmission of the information, data storage and presentation of that information.

9.7.1.1 Collection of Data

The data collecting stage is the initial step in the data flow, and it has a significant impact on the future stages, which include network access, data storage, energy usage and system architecture, among others. Depending on whether the infrastructure is

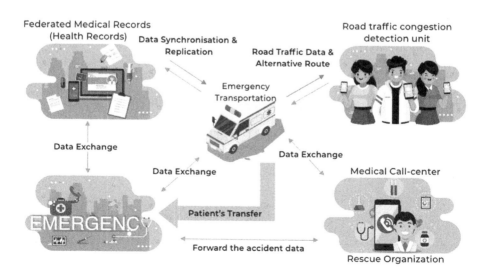

FIGURE 9.4 Important areas of IoT analytics in medicine.

stationary or movable, the data gathering approach can be a combination of random sampling and continuous sampling. A more modern sensing technology, based on RFID and WSN, has been developed and implemented, but a new one, participatory sensing, has evolved in recent years. It accomplishes this by taking advantage of the ubiquity of sensor-rich, internet-enabled smartphones, as well as the mobility of the people, to deliver a level of finer, more granular sensing that was before unattainable. Extending participatory sensing technologies presents us with a slew of benefits, including the elimination of hardware costs and the ability to conduct sensing on demand. Although the basic question of whether participatory sensing would produce accurate data remains unanswered, there is some optimism. The incorporation of several incentives and competitions to persuade more persons to join is an alternative method of dealing with the dilemma.

9.7.1.2 Management and Preprocessing of Datasets

In order to generate valuable information and intelligence from raw data, it is necessary to process it before it can be used to generate that information. The use of event detection from long-duration time series data is typically recommended when it gets to this stage since it allows for more accurate event identification. It is essential that algorithms be flexible and resilient in order to deal with data from a wide range of temporal and spatial dimensions and time scales. If you want to provide a complete interpretation of the results, it is recommended that you employ advanced computational approaches, for example, evolutionary algorithms, neural networks and genetic algorithms to convert raw data into information. While data retention will remain as crucial as it is now, the ability to use data to preserve and research historical records will become increasingly important as time progresses.

9.7.1.3 Interpretation of Datasets

The ultimate purpose of a data-centric Internet of Things architecture is to transform raw sensor data into data that can be used to generate insight and knowledge. Today's increasingly efficient computer hardware and digital new technologies make things easier to do, allowing for more intuitive and open knowledge display to users. Among the most contemporary technologies available, touch screen displays allow users to navigate data by simply touching it. Touch screen displays are becoming increasingly popular. By allowing data to be reflected in a more precise manner, 3D displays help to improve data representation [36].

9.7.2 Cloud-Centric IoT Platform

When combined with smart city technology, the cloud-centric IoT design is meant to blend IoT features and smart city capabilities while maximizing the benefits of cloud computing. Sensors connected to the network generate data in this system, which is subsequently kept in cloud storage by software engineers who are developing framework-supporting applications to support the system. For their part, data mining and deep learning specialists are employed to translate raw data into facts and understanding. When it comes to cloud computing, there are a variety of

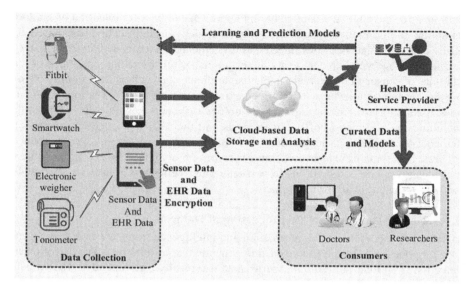

FIGURE 9.5   Systematic overview of cloud-centric IoT platform [37].

services available, comprising infrastructure-as-a-service (IaaS), platform-as-a-service (PaaS), and software-as-a-service (SaaS), to name a few. Consequently, data acquired by sensors, software that maintains the device and algorithms that process the data would be safeguarded from being accessed by the general public through applications that are not protected. Using cloud storage and computation as the foundation of an Internet of Things architecture, all aspects of distributed computing will be integrated while providing scalable storage and processing resources. See Figure 9.5 for an overview.

9.7.3   NETWORK-CENTRIC IoT

It is possible to implement an internet-based or object-based network-centric IoT architecture in either of the two types described above. The internet-based system will place a strong emphasis on the internet and the use of internet networks as the primary means of data transport, with the internet serving as a critical component of the design. Smart objects can be used to create object-based designs, although they are not required. In this network-centric Internet of Things approach, the networking infrastructure serves as the network kernel. IoT designs that are network-centric, like earlier architectures, have a major emphasis on sensor types, addressing devices, networking models and quality of service operations [37].

9.7.3.1   Sensing Paradigm

RFID, WSN (Wireless Sensor Network), and crowd sourcing are the sensing paradigms that are currently most commonly used. RFID tags are used to categorize things and behaviours based on their radio frequency identification (RFID) tags. When the reader asks a query of the symbols, they respond by revealing their unique IDs, which are subsequently relayed to the reader by the reader. Given the rising use of RFID technology in the transportation and access control industries, the use of RFID in a smart city is a logical extension of this trend. In terms of sensing paradigms, WSN is the principal representation, and it comprises four important activities: gathering valuable input from external fields, evaluating that input, decoding that input, and communicating the results. Sensor properties such as improved power, compactness and reliability, as well as cheaper production costs, are now widely used. Other advantages include decreased manufacturing costs. Due to the advancement of sensors in terms of size, dependability and power, sensor networks such as sensor networks are becoming increasingly significant. As a modern sensing model, crowd sourcing is a sensing as a participatory internet-enabled process in which everyone's smartphones are interested. Our crowd sensing technologies have been improved to the point where we are now able to deliver sensing capabilities that were previously unavailable due to their reduced time and space granularity. Because smartphones now have a higher ability to view the world and the amount of people who inhabit it, future devices will incorporate more sensors.

9.7.3.2   Addressing Scheme
Using this strategy, we are primarily concerned with giving each artifact a unique identity. In addition to allowing for the primary recognition and differentiation of all instruments, it also allows for their connection to and monitoring. With the rising number of devices and networks, we would design the network in such a way that it would not be a significant obstacle to its overall performance. IPv4 has not yet displayed any signs of vulnerability and continues to be the most frequently used protocol on the internet. However, in a short period of time, the address space would be almost completely depleted. Because it has a far bigger address space than its predecessor, IPv4, the new internet protocol version 6 is an excellent replacement for IPv4. It provides unique addresses for all computers on the earth. Furthermore, IPv6 contains characteristics that are compatible with a wide range of formats and networking networks, but it is still simple to use on devices that have been refused access to the internet protocol version 6. In a network-centric AIoT design, the Zigbee protocol adds another reliable addressing scheme for IoT devices, making it a complete package. There are three pure addresses associated with each Zigbee machine: a permanent 64-bit MAC address, a 16-bit network address and a string of names that can be used for a variety of purposes [38]. The MAC address of a Zigbee machine is 64 bits long, but the network address of a Zigbee network is 16 bits long and is established by the Zigbee network supervisor or the router that manages the network. This addressing method is well-suited to the complexity and routing requirements of Zigbee schemes.

9.7.3.3   Connectivity Model
It was the TCP/IP architecture that laid the foundation for the development of the internet. Because the TCP/IP layers have been integrated into a layered configuration, WSNs can employ this architecture to meet their own standards, such as low-power

service, network scalability, and minimal resource consumption, among others. A large number of networking layers existed in the first-generation TCP/IP architecture, with each layer serving as a resource for the layer below it. The physical layer, the MAC layer, the network layer, the transport layer and the application layer are the layers that make up the OSI model. When it comes to WSN implementations, the same architecture is used.

9.7.3.4   Quality of Service (QoS) Mechanism

To accommodate the variety of protocol (wired and wireless) and sensor types, an Internet of Things architecture must incorporate a number of heterogeneous networking networks, network operation and quality of service considerations. For example, multiple IoT applications for the Padova smart city project, each having its own set of characteristics, as well as its own traffic and delay necessities, network kinds and energy source. This is an excellent illustration of the various structures of an Internet of Things architecture. In order to better understand this term, consider two types of network traffic: elastic throughput and elastic delay tolerant traffic, and inelastic bandwidth and inelastic delay tolerant traffic.

The rapid evolution of wearable biosensors and wireless communication technologies has resulted in the development of a variety of smart healthcare solutions for the real-time monitoring of patient health. These systems, on the other hand, contain a slew of security weaknesses such as, a password guessing attack on IoT devices can negotiate them, resulting in the breach of health data privacy. After providing the summary of the security concerns associated with the IoT in healthcare, this article examines the security flaws associated with password creation and proposes a method for evaluating password strength that takes into account users' personal information to ensure that passwords are strong. The next section highlights the security and privacy concerns that must be considered in AIoT healthcare.

9.8   SECURITY AND PRIVACY REQUIREMENTS OF AIOT HEALTHCARE

Clinical diagnostics and emergency medical response to patients in medical care facilities as well as at home through remote medical procedures are among the services and applications provided. Patients' data is kept in a data centre or database that may be accessed through the internet.

The development of a extensive range of IoT devices and applications in the healthcare sector has recently been observed. These devices handle sensitive and private information, such as personal health information, and may be targeted by cyber criminals to steal it. Understanding the characteristics and principles of security requirements in the healthcare Internet of Things is critical. We examined previously published studies on the security requirements of IoT-based healthcare applications in this study. The study's findings are intended to be useful to a wide range of communities, including researchers, information technology engineers, health care professionals, and government officials dealing with Internet of Things and healthcare technologies, among others. This work serves as inspiration for future research and the development of a resilient Internet of Things-based healthcare system.

Additional benefits include access to various healthcare specialists, such as those that conduct medical diagnoses in order to treat patients, through cloud computing. These facilities are rapidly altering the traditional nature of patient care, increasing the efficiency and effectiveness of medical processes while also lowering costs [39]. Aside from that, these healthcare applications make it possible to monitor patients from a distance using smart devices such as smartphones and wearable sensors. The impact and influence of a range of AIoT-H implementations on a variety of AIoT applications may be of particular interest to academics with a vested interest in the issue.

The key tasks of a cloud data center include data storage, data management, and data security protection, to name a few. In the field of data storage, there are many different functions, including video data storage, picture data storage, structured data storage, and semi-structured data storage, among others. Database administration encompasses the processes of data aggregation and management as well as the analysis and presentation of data. Data security protection is largely concerned with the encryption and isolation of sensitive data, as well as access control, rights management, backup recovery, and audit logs, amongst other aspects of information technology [39].

Healthcare applications that are safe and secure are necessary to improve patients' well-being while also taking into account the security and privacy concerns that they bring into patients' lives, as well as other implications such as privacy violations and financial risks [40] (see Figure 9.6). By digging into the various components of the application architecture, the chapter examines the privacy and security concerns connected with IoT healthcare applications.

For instance, smartphones and wearable sensor devices with remote monitoring capabilities are examples of such gadgets. The procedures of remote patient monitoring and alarm systems are supported by healthcare services and software, respectively. Because the information provided by these procedures is considered sensitive, the information generated by these processes is the most valued benefit of these applications. The rationale for this is that it has a direct impact on the well-being and safety of patients and their families. It is always dangerous to compromise sensitive data because it has a substantial influence on the privacy and security of a complete system as well as its stakeholders. Furthermore, the confidentiality and accessibility of these data must be safeguarded against disclosure. Furthermore, sensitive data should be safeguarded in order to prevent illegal access as well as other dangers and threats from occurring. The volume of data generated by sensor devices, as well as the continual connectivity between the devices in the system, make these sections of an AIoT ecosystem particularly challenging and time-consuming. Recent years have seen a collaboration between healthcare professionals and application developers to develop secure IoT healthcare applications to address these issues [41].

9.9 CONCLUSION AND FUTURE WORK

The major goals of the ehealth is to make healthcare services available to patients from the comfort of their own homes, particularly through the use of AI and the IoTs. In order to do this, AI apps are often designed to save money while also inspiring patients at home, resulting in higher patient involvement. Improved health promotion

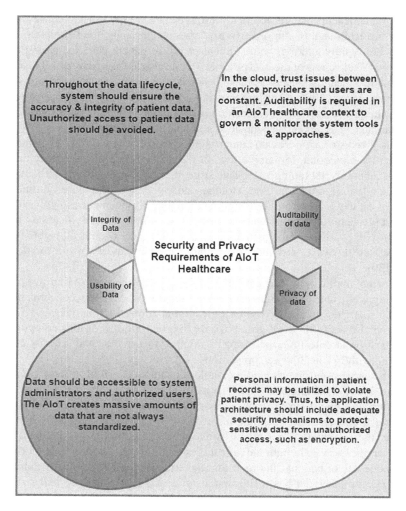

FIGURE 9.6   Security and privacy requirements of AIoT healthcare.

and a more enjoyable lifestyle will arise as a result of this for everyone. According to the conclusions of this study, the IoT in the medical sector is still in its infancy. In a number of sub-fields, the utilization-limiting application has been implemented, and it appears to have placed a major pressure on the healthcare system in general. More significantly, as the number of medical AIoT studies and research areas increased in 2018, the number of studies on this issue will grow in the future, leading in more research fields participating.

Using the IoT, information from multiple sensory elements may be communicated successfully to an IoT hub or control center, where it might be utilised for monitoring, diagnosis and assistance as well as intelligent decision-making. Information gathered from patient, medical equipment, hospitals, ambulances, recovery centres, nursing homes and other facilities can be used to help construct smart settings for the elderly and infirm. Monitoring patients' vital signs on a regular basis, appointment scheduling, after-care assistance, geriatric assistance, disease diagnosis, vulnerability analysis and priority management are all made possible in these smart environments. If efficient cloud-based solutions are not incorporated into IoT-enabled healthcare, all of these systems will stay regional and isolated, as they have done in the past. These modest, isolated IoT solutions can be integrated into a completely intelligent healthcare infrastructure through the utilisation of cloud-computing services. The IoT and cloud-based healthcare systems can evaluate changes on a bigger scale and predict epidemics, healthcare crises, system limitations and future requirements in real time, allowing the healthcare system to be better prepared to address emergencies. Patient monitoring, post-procedure observation, patient prioritizing, diagnostics, support, vulnerability analysis, threat forecasting and future requirements are all possible with joint IoT and cloud-based solutions.

Patients, healthcare professionals and insurance companies all play important roles in the healthcare sector, which is a broad and diversified industry encompassing an extensive range of performers, including patients, healthcare professionals and insurance firms. While artificial intelligence is not yet widely used in many medical sub-fields, it is gaining ground in those areas. Regardless of whether AIoT, healthcare and medicine have significant overlap, AIoT has not been fully accepted in some areas due to the interdisciplinary nature of the subject matter. This investigation may be of interest to scholars who are concerned with understanding this occurrence. Depending on the circumstances, this goal will be achieved qualitatively through interviews with specific demographics or quantitatively through book searches.

REFERENCES

[1] Fahad Taha Al-Dhief, Nurul Mu'azzah Abdul Latiff, Nik Noordini Nik Abd Malik, Naseer Sabri Salim, Marina Mat Baki, Musatafa Abbas Abbood Albadr, and Mazin Abed Mohammed. A survey of voice pathology surveillance systems based on internet of things and machine learning algorithms. *IEEE Access*, 8:64514–64533, 2020.

[2] Maria Cvach. Monitor alarm fatigue: an integrative review. *Biomedical instrumentation & technology*, 46(4):268–277, 2012.

[3] Barbara J Drew, Patricia Harris, Jessica K Zègre-Hemsey, Tina Mammone, Daniel Schindler, Rebeca Salas-Boni, Yong Bai, Adelita Tinoco, Quan Ding, and Xiao Hu. Insights into the problem of alarm fatigue with physiologic monitor devices: a comprehensive observational study of consecutive intensive care unit patients. *PloS one*, 9(10):e110274, 2014.

[4] Kelly Creighton Graham and Maria Cvach. Monitor alarm fatigue: standardizing use of physiological monitors and decreasing nuisance alarms. *American Journal of Critical Care*, 19(1):28–34, 2010.

[5] Jeffrey M Rothschild, Christopher P Landrigan, John W Cronin, Rainu Kaushal, Steven W Lockley, Elisabeth Burdick, Peter H Stone, Craig M Lilly, Joel T Katz, Charles A Czeisler, et al. The critical care safety study: The incidence and nature of adverse events and serious medical errors in intensive care. *Read Online: Critical Care Medicine| Society of Critical Care Medicine*, 33(8):1694–1700, 2005.

[6] Pascale Carayon and Ays¸e P Gürses. A human factors engineering conceptual framework of nursing workload and patient safety in intensive care units. *Intensive and Critical Care Nursing*, 21(5):284–301, 2005.

[7] Pascale Carayon. Human factors of complex sociotechnical systems. *Applied ergonomics*, 37(4):525–535, 2006.

[8] Shih-Hao Chang, Rui-Dong Chiang, Shih-Jung Wu, and Wei-Ting Chang. A context-aware, interactive m-health system for diabetics. *IT professional*, 18(3):14–22, 2016.

[9] Jingyu Zhang, Siqi Zhong, Jin Wang, Xiaofeng Yu, and Osama Alfarraj. A storage optimization scheme for blockchain transaction databases. *COMPUTER SYSTEMS SCIENCE AND ENGINEERING*, 36(3):521–535, 2021.

[10] YIN Yuehong, Yan Zeng, Xing Chen, and Yuanjie Fan. The internet of things in healthcare: An overview. *Journal of Industrial Information Integration*, 1:3–13, 2016.

[11] Cristian F Pasluosta, Heiko Gassner, Juergen Winkler, Jochen Klucken, and Bjoern M Eskofier. An emerging era in the management of Parkinson's disease: wearable technologies and the internet of things. *IEEE journal of biomedical and health informatics*, 19(6):1873–1881, 2015.

[12] Georg Wolgast, Casimir Ehrenborg, Alexander Israelsson, Jakob Helander, Edvard Johansson, and Hampus Manefjord. Wireless body area network for heart attack detection [education corner]. *IEEE antennas and propagation magazine*, 58(5):84–92, 2016.

[13] Antonio J Jara, Miguel A Zamora-Izquierdo, and Antonio F Skarmeta. Interconnection framework for mhealth and remote monitoring based on the internet of things. *IEEE Journal on Selected Areas in Communications*, 31(9):47–65, 2013.

[14] Mahmoud Elkhodr, Seyed Shahrestani, and Hon Cheung. Internet of things applications: current and future development. In *Innovative Research and Applications in Next-Generation High Performance Computing*, pages 397–427. IGI Global, 2016.

[15] Haipeng Peng, Ye Tian, Jürgen Kurths, Lixiang Li, Yixian Yang, and Daoshun Wang. Secure and energy-efficient data transmission system based on chaotic compressive sensing in body-to-body networks. *IEEE transactions on biomedical circuits and systems*, 11(3):558–573, 2017.

[16] Michelle A Cretikos, Rinaldo Bellomo, Ken Hillman, Jack Chen, Simon Finfer, and Arthas Flabouris. Respiratory rate: the neglected vital sign. *Medical Journal of Australia*, 188(11):657–659, 2008.

[17] V Jagadeeswari, V Subramaniyaswamy, R Logesh, and Varadarajan Vijayakumar. A study on medical internet of things and big data in personalized healthcare system. *Health information science and systems*, 6(1):1–20, 2018.

[18] Renan CA Alves, Lucas Batista Gabriel, Bruno Trevizan de Oliveira, Cintia Borges Margi, and Fabíola Car- valho Lopes dos Santos. Assisting physical (hydro) therapy with wireless sensors networks. *IEEE Internet of Things Journal*, 2(2):113–120, 2015.

[19] Ji Li, Ping Wang, and Youliang Xu. Prognostic value of programmed cell death ligand 1 expression in patients with head and neck cancer: A systematic review and meta-analysis. *PLOS ONE*, 12(6):1–16, 06 2017.

[20] Arthur Gatouillat, Youakim Badr, Bertrand Massot, and Ervin Sejdic´. Internet of medical things: A review of recent contributions dealing with cyber-physical systems in medicine. *IEEE internet of things journal*, 5(5):3810–3822, 2018.

[21] SM Riazul Islam, Daehan Kwak, MD Humaun Kabir, Mahmud Hossain, and Kyung-Sup Kwak. The internet of things for health care: a comprehensive survey. *IEEE access*, 3:678–708, 2015.

[22] Dimiter V Dimitrov. Medical internet of things and big data in healthcare. *Healthcare informatics research*, 22(3):156, 2016.

[23] Stephanie B Baker, Wei Xiang, and Ian Atkinson. Internet of things for smart healthcare: Technologies, challenges, and opportunities. *IEEE Access*, 5:26521–26544, 2017.

[24] P Yang, J Qi, G Min, and L Xu. Advanced internet of things for personalised healthcare system: A survey. *Pervasive and Mobile Computing*, 41:132–149, 2017.

[25] Bahar Farahani, Farshad Firouzi, Victor Chang, Mustafa Badaroglu, Nicholas Constant, and Kunal Mankodiya. Towards fog-driven iot ehealth: Promises and challenges of iot in medicine and healthcare. *Future Generation Computer Systems*, 78:659–676, 2018.

[26] L Minh Dang, Md Piran, Dongil Han, Kyungbok Min, Hyeonjoon Moon, et al. A survey on internet of things and cloud computing for healthcare. *Electronics*, 8(7):768, 2019.

[27] Hossein Ahmadi, Goli Arji, Leila Shahmoradi, Reza Safdari, Mehrbakhsh Nilashi, and Mojtaba Alizadeh. The application of internet of things in healthcare: a systematic literature review and classification. *Universal Access in the Information Society*, 18(4):837–869, 2019.

[28] Shah Nazir, Yasir Ali, Naeem Ullah, and Iván García-Magariño. Internet of things for healthcare using effects of mobile computing: a systematic literature review. *Wireless Communications and Mobile Computing*, 2019, 2019.

[29] Itamir de Morais Barroca Filho and Gibeon Soares de Aquino Junior. Iot-based healthcare applications: a review. In *International conference on computational science and its applications*, pages 47–62. Springer, 2017.

[30] Ammar Awad Mutlag, Mohd Khanapi Abd Ghani, Net al Arunkumar, Mazin Abed Mohammed, and Othman Mohd. Enabling technologies for fog computing in healthcare iot systems. *Future Generation Computer Systems*, 90:62–78, 2019.

[31] Noemi Scarpato, Alessandra Pieroni, Luca Di Nunzio, and Francesca Fallucchi. E-health-IoT universe: A review. *management*, 21(44):46, 2017.

[32] Amit Kumar Podder, Abdullah Al Bukhari, Sayemul Islam, Sujon Mia, Mazin Abed Mohammed, Nallapa- neni Manoj Kumar, Korhan Cengiz, and Karrar Hameed Abdulkareem. Iot based smart agrotech system for verification of urban farming parameters. *Microprocessors and Microsystems*, 82:104025, 2021.

[33] Anil Pise, Hima Vadapalli, and Ian Sanders. Facial emotion recognition using temporal relational network: an application to e-learning. *Multimedia Tools and Applications*, pages 1–21, 2020.

[34] Jun Qi, Po Yang, Geyong Min, Oliver Amft, Feng Dong, and Lida Xu. Advanced internet of things for personalised healthcare systems: A survey. *Pervasive and Mobile Computing*, 41:132–149, 2017.

[35] Jiong Jin, Jayavardhana Gubbi, Slaven Marusic, and Marimuthu Palaniswami. An information framework for creating a smart city through internet of things. *IEEE Internet of Things journal*, 1(2):112–121, 2014.

[36] Wangdong Yang, Kenli Li, Zeyao Mo, and Keqin Li. Performance optimization using partitioned spmv on gpus and multicore cpus. *IEEE Transactions on Computers*, 64(9):2623–2636, 2014.

[37] Jun Du, Chunxiao Jiang, Erol Gelenbe, Lei Xu, Jianhua Li, and Yong Ren. Distributed data privacy preservation in iot applications. *IEEE Wireless Communications*, 25(6):68–76, 2018.

[38] Ethan Perez, Harm de Vries, Florian Strub, Vincent Dumoulin, and Aaron Courville. Learning visual reasoning without strong priors. *arXiv preprint arXiv:1707.03017*, 2017.

[39] Daojing He, Ran Ye, Sammy Chan, Mohsen Guizani, and Yanping Xu. Privacy in the internet of things for smart healthcare. *IEEE Communications Magazine*, 56(4):38–44, 2018.

[40] Suvini P Amaraweera and Malka N Halgamuge. Internet of things in the healthcare sector: overview of security and privacy issues. *Security, privacy and trust in the IoT environment*, pages 153–179, 2019.

[41] Hai Tao, Md Zakirul Alam Bhuiyan, Ahmed N Abdalla, Mohammad Mehedi Hassan, Jasni Mohamad Zain, and Thaier Hayajneh. Secured data collection with hardware-based ciphers for iot-based healthcare. *IEEE Internet of Things Journal*, 6(1):410–420, 2018.

10 An IoT-Based Moving Vehicle Healthcare Service

Vandana Roy,[1] Hemant Amhia,[2] Shailja Shukla,[2] and A. K. Wadhwani[3]
[1] Gyan Ganga Institute of Technology and Science, Jabalpur, Madhya Pradesh, India
[2] Jabalpur Engineering College, Jabalpur, Madhya Pradesh, India
[3] Madhav Institute of Technology and Science (MITS), Gwalior Madhya Pradesh, India

CONTENTS

DOI: 10.1201/9781003145035-10

10.1   INTRODUCTION

It is possible to exchange data between physical objects via the Internet of Things (IoT). All of these IoT technologies have evolved over time, including sensors, machine learning, real-time analytics and embedded systems. There are many devices in the smart hospital concept that use fixed or wireless internet to control. The task at hand can be accomplished by using smart devices to collect and share data. Smart cities, cars, devices, entertainment systems, homes and connected healthcare are all benefiting from IoT applications. It is essential to use a variety of sensors and medical devices as well as AI, diagnostics and high-end imaging devices when implementing the IoT in healthcare settings. In both old and new industries and societies, these devices have a positive impact on productivity and quality of life.

Prior to the invention of the wheel, primitive man existed in separation from supplementary tribes and societies. They could only get to work if it was a short walk. The advent of the wheel ushered in a new era in early man's development. Prehistoric man evolved into a mannered, civilized individual over time, and the wheel's design was refined as well. There has been a rise in the figure of recorded motor automobiles in Delhi from 525,000 to 864,000 between 2014 and 2016, which has directed to an upsurge in the number of accidents and, consequently, the number of casualties. However, according to India Spends 2015 report on traffic-related deaths, motor vehicle accidents registered for 83% of all road traffic-associated deaths in 2015. There is no human intervention in the data transfer through the internet as a consequence of the (IoT) Internet of Things. During the COVID 19 pandemic, this technology is soaring in healthcare monitoring. In today's world, many people are dying as a result of misinformation about their health. By using sensors, this technology can quickly alert the user of any health concerns. All COVID 19 patient-related data is stored in the cloud, which can aid in providing the proper level of attention. This technology is able to monitor a person's daily activities and alert them if they are experiencing a health issue.

Having the proper medical equipment is a necessity for a successful medical procedure. The IoT is well-suited to both performing successful operations and assessing the results of those operations. The application of IoT during the COVID 19 pandemic progresses patient care. It is possible to perform real-time monitoring with IoT and to save lives from a variety of conditions, including diabetes, heart failure, asthma attacks and hypertension. Using a smartphone, smart medical devices are able to transmit the necessary health data to the physician. These devices also monitor oxygen, blood pressure, weight and sugar levels.

10.2   GOAL OF THE RESEARCH WORK

There are many factors that can cause fatal car accidents, and this study aims to address those issues while also providing safety measures. Traveling to far-flung destinations and reducing the amount of time it takes is impossible without transportation. Although the number of vehicles on the road is steadily increasing, this must be taken into account. There are measures in place after an accident, as well as measures to prevent them from happening again. An investigation into car accidents has resulted from this study.

- Seat belts are treated as an afterthought.
- DWI (driving while intoxicated).
- Drowsy driving, which results in a driver's inattention.

10.3 OBJECTIVE

The following outcomes are anticipated as a result of this plan:

- Do not start the engine unless the seat belts are securely fastened.
- Ensure that the driver is not intoxicated by deploying a gas senor. Only when the motorist is sober will the engine start.
- Eye-blink feelers are connected in the automobile to guarantee that the motorist is not sleepy.
- Proximity sensors are used to avoid a collision by detecting any obstacles that may be ahead of the vehicle.
- After a crash, a GPS-founded attentive arrangement is attached to pinpoint the exact location of the exhausted flatcar and send a notification to the appropriate party. A vibration sensor picks up on the accident.

10.4 EXISTING WORK DONE

A Raspberry Pi-based handling chip is used by [1] to create a monocular vision, self-sufficient auto model. An ultrasonic sensor and a high-definition camera were used to provide the car with basic evidence from the existing realism. To avoid human error, the vehicle is capable of accomplishing the given task safely and thoroughly. Several current calculations, such as route documentation and impairment position, are associated to provide critical regulation to the automobile. The chapter implements the arrangement on a Raspberry Pi, because of its ethical processor. An accelerometer-grounded arrangement for motorist protection was projected by [2]. For quick access to the control and event discovery, this framework makes use of Raspberry Pi (ARM11). In the event of an emergency, a message is sent to the appropriate establishments so that they can react rapidly and efficiently to save, support and mitigate harm. The proposed model is incompetent and incomplete because it only includes one element and flouts the supplementary incurable grounds. For the vehicles, crash avoidance arrangement [3] projected an effective approach to identify the obstacles in its front and blind spots. With a beeper and an LED symbol, the driver is alerted to a decreasing distance between their vehicle and an obstacle. Using an ultrasonic sensor, a vehicle's ultrasonic system can tell whether an object is moving or not. It's a great tool for spotting other vehicles, motorcycles, bikes and pedestrians who cross in front of you on the side of the road. The chapter uses a Raspberry Pi microcomputer to run the proposed system, but it has a limited performance out-of-the-box.

It was proposed by [4] to incorporate an alcohol detector into an effective vehicle collision aversion framework. Using this system, the driver can be alerted to the amount of alcohol they've consumed, and an LCD screen displays this information. A buzzer is used to alert the driver of his or her own situation, as well as to frighten others in the vicinity [5]. The driver in an abnormally high state of drowsiness will

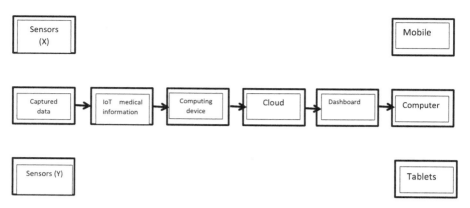

FIGURE 10.1   IoT implementation process chart.

not be able to start a vehicle because the flinch outline will be disabled. Ironically, this tactic mechanism is to make the driver more aware of his own condition while also intimidating him into doing anything about it. The concept is novel, but it's not practical.

Doctors, surgeons, and patients will benefit greatly from IoT systems that take on new challenges in the medical field. Step-by-step instructions are provided for an efficient IoT implementation. Figure 10.1 depicts the IoT process flow in the healthcare industry.

10.5   HEALTHCARE IOT SERVICES

It was previously impossible for doctors to make real-time analysis of a patient's condition because of the lack of IoT technology. Healthcare facilities have been able to serve a larger number of people at a lower cost because of this initiative. Patient-doctor communication has become more dependable and simple thanks to the use of big data and cloud computing. As a result, there was a higher level of patient participation in treatment as well as a lower financial burden on the patient. Health and fitness management, sickness judgment, individual repair for children and the aging and chronic disease monitoring are all examples of HIoT applications that have been influenced by the Internet of Things (IoT) in recent years. It has been broken down into two main categories, namely facilities and solicitations, in order to better understand these applications. Health-related IoT devices can be classified into two categories: those used in the development of new medical devices and those used for monitoring and diagnosing existing conditions.

10.6   AMENITIES

The healthcare industry has been transformed by new services and concepts that address a wide range of healthcare issues. With the increasing demand for healthcare and the advancement of technology, more services are being added on a daily basis. These are now an essential part of the HIoT system design process. In a HIoT environment, each service offers a variety of healthcare options. You won't find a single other definition for these terms or services. The applications of HIoT systems are what make them stand out. Consequently, it is difficult to formulate a general definition for each concept. However, in the following section, specifics of the most commonly applied IoT healthcare facilities have been designated.

10.6.1 Assisted Living in a More Natural Setting

It is a special division of artificial intelligence (AI) that uses IoT to assist the elderly and is called AAL (ambient assisted living). One of the main goals of AAL is to make it easier and safer for the elderly to remain in their own homes for as long as possible. In the event of a medical emergency, AAL offers a method for practical-time checking of these subjects and ensuring that they obtain humanoid service-comparable support. Using progressive AI skills, large statistics study, machine learning and their application in healthcare businesses, this is possible. There are three main areas of AAL that have been studied by researchers: action acknowledgment, atmosphere acknowledgment and dynamic observing. Activity recognition, on the other hand, drew the most attention because it focuses on noticing possible intimidations or emergency healthiness circumstances that could harm elderly patients. Abundant trainings have documented the use of IoT in AAL. Health care solutions for the elderly were proposed by [6]. The writer intended a segmental building for AAL safety, automation and communication. Communication protocols used throughout enactment included RFID and NFC. Using a closed-ring communication facility, this device connects the patient through the healthcare benefactors. Advanced IoT-founded AAL systems can be built on top of this protocol, which was developed from the aforementioned architecture. Recently, in an effort to assist the elderly with enduring circumstances and additional possible health crises, the authors have developed an emergency detector. As a result, caregivers were alerted in the event of an emergency. With the help of assistive robots, IoT-founded healthcare arrangements are currently capable to monitor inside air quality. Alerts are sent to caregivers if the air quality drops below a predetermined standard level. [7] proposes a protected, exposed and flexible stage for AAL based on an IoT-founded entryway integrated with cloud computing. The gateway was instrumental in resolving a number of IoT-related security, data storage and interoperability problems.

10.6.2 Mobile Internet of Things

Patients' health data and other physiological conditions can be tracked using mobile calculating, sensors, communication skills and cloud calculating. An effectual internet-grounded healthcare facility can be provided through PANs, 4G and 5G. It has been made easier for healthcare practitioners to contact the subject's statistics, analyze and quickly offer action thanks to the use of mobile devices. The use of mobile computing in healthcare has been the subject of several studies [8]. Diabetic patients with low blood sugar can now have their glucose levels monitored using an m-IoT-based system developed by [9]. At the same time, an "AMBRO" HIoT system for fall detection and heart rate control was developed in another study. In addition, a GPS module built into the device could help locate the patients. When a patient's heart rate exceeds 60–100 beats per minute, an IoT-founded practical-time observing arrangement is able to detect an irregularity in the heart action and alert the subject. In an m-IoT system, it's critical to protect the privacy and security of users and their data.

10.6.3 DEVICES THAT CAN BE WORN ON THE BODY

With the help of wearable devices, healthcare specialists and patients can deal with a wide range of health issues for less money. A variety of sensors can be integrated into wearable accessories, such as a wristwatch, wristband, necklet, shoe, bag, top and so on, to create these noninvasive devices. The sensor attached collects information about the patient's health and the surrounding environment. The server/databases are then notified of this information. Mobile health applications allow some wearables to communicate with smartphones. The use of these wearable devices and mobile computing in real-time monitoring has been documented in the literature [10]. With IoT-enabled wearable systems, patients' vital information such as electrocardiogram and electromyogram signals could also be extracted from their bio signals [11]. The computational power of these wearable devices is boosted thanks to their connection to a mobile app. The collected data can then be processed and visualized using the application. Figure 10.2 shows various types of IoT devices which can be attached on the human body for analysis.

10.6.4 PROVIDERS OF COMMUNITY-BASED HEALTHCARE

Health monitoring in the community is done by building a healthcare system that spans a small area, for example, a reserved hospital or an apartment complex. This type of health monitoring is referred to as community-based healthcare monitoring.

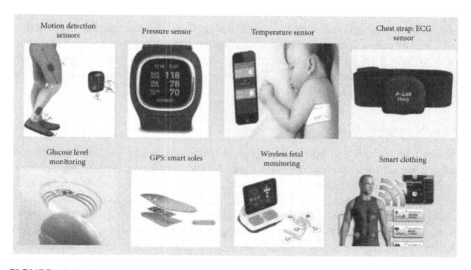

FIGURE 10.2 IoT sensors applied on the human body.

Multiple networks are linked together to form a community network that can provide a collaborative service. An Internet-of-Things (IoT)-founded supportive medicinal system was established in [12] to offer remote healthcare observing. Various methods of authentication and authorization were used to ensure the safety of the network connection. Another study proposed a "virtual hospital" for a local medical network. This made it possible to provide medical care to those in need even from a distance. [12] makes the case for establishing a resident health network. Patients' medical records are included in a four level organizational outline that was intended herein. The wellbeing centers in the area can use this information to give correct medicinal guidance to patients who live there.

10.6.5 THE STUDY OF THE MIND

To use computing in a way similar to how the human brain does it, we say we're using "cognitive calculating". IoT measures are now equipped with sensors having the latest developments in sensor technology and artificial intelligence that can solve problems like the human intelligence can do. Using cognitive computing in an IoT system can help uncover patterns in a large amount of data [13]. The sensor's ability to process healthcare data and automatically adapt to the environment is also improved. All sensors work together with other smart gadgets in a cognitive IoT network to provide effective health services. Patients' data can be effectively analyzed and treated with the help of cognitive computing, which is incorporated into an IoT system. In addition, it makes it easier to get help in the event of a disease outbreak. Patients' health data can be detected, recorded, and analyzed with the help of the cognitive data transmission method proposed by Kumar et al. A patient's vital information is transmitted with the utmost urgency in an emergency situation [14].

10.6.6 UNWANTED SIDE EFFECTS OF A MEDICINE

As a side effect, an ADR (adverse drug reaction) can be described. There is a chance that the reaction will happen either after a sole dosage or completed time. Adverse reactions from taking two different medicines at once may also contribute to this. Antibiotic-related adverse reactions (ADR) are not influenced by the category of medication or the illness being treated, but rather by the individual patient. In an IoT- founded ADR scheme, each medicine is identified at the patient's terminal by a unique identifier/barcode [15]. It is possible to use a pharmaceutical intelligent information system to verify the medication's compatibility with the patient's body. Each patient's ehealth records are used to store their allergy profile in the information system. A medication's suitability for a patient is determined by examining the patient's allergy profile and other relevant health data.

10.6.7 BLOCKCHAIN

A HIoT network relies heavily on the distribution of statistics between medicinal planners and healthcare workers. However, data fragmentation is a major issue when it comes to secure data sharing. There may be a break in info between healthcare benefactors who are linked to the same patient as a consequence of data disintegration. Treatment can be hampered by a lack of information. Healthcare centers can use blockchain technology to resolve the issue of records disintegration and establish a link between data repositories in the network. [16] Additional security measures are in place to protect sensitive medical information and to enhance patient-doctor communication. Qualitative research in healthcare is made easier with the help of blockchain technology. There are three possible reasons for the secure transmission provided by blockchain technology. A "ledger" that can be edited and measured by individuals is the first feature. It prevents any tampering with the data once it has been entered into the ledger. Additional rules govern how each transaction in the ledger is recorded. First of all, because the blockchain is a decentralized technology, it is able to operate simultaneously from a variety of devices. Using smart contracts, blockchain complies with the rules of agreement and data exchange. The smart contract controls access to the blockchain-stored electronic medical records (EMRs) and maintains a user's identity. This means that doctors can only access EMRs to which they have been granted access. A blockchain-based application termed as HDG (healthcare data gateway) was developed by authors to give patients control over the sharing of their medical records. Using this method, patients can maintain full control over their personal data while still adhering to the policy's strict confidentiality requirements [17].

10.6.8 INFORMATION FOR PARENTS CONCERNED ABOUT THE HEALTH OF THEIR CHILDREN

The idea of disseminating information about children's health is known as "CHI." To do this, we wish to educate and empower children and parents about their child's complete health, which includes nutritional values, emotional/mental state and behaviour. This is the primary objective of the CHI. The Internet of Things has been used to construct a platform that can be used to monitor and control the health of a child. For monitoring a child's mental and physical healthiness, there has been formed an Internet of Things (IoT) outline [18]. It's also possible to take immediate action in an emergency by working with doctors and parents. It measures five different aspects of the user's health: height, temperature, saturation percentage, weightiness and heart degree. The app makes this info obtainable to clinicians and other health care providers. Teachers and parents could use an mhealth provision to screen children's nourishment habits, according to [19]. The app was used to ensure that the children's nutritional needs were met.

10.7 APPLICATION OF IOT

There are a variety of IoT-based applications that can be developed using the HIoft services/concepts. Researchers in these fields have come up with a slew of ideas aimed at improving all of us. Applications, on the other hand, focus on end users, whereas concepts cater more to developers. Wearable sensors, portable gadgets and medical devices have become more affordable and user-friendly thanks to the rapid development of IoT technology. It is possible to collect patient data, diagnose diseases and keep tabs on their health.

10.7.1 ECG Detection and Monitoring

The depolarization of the atria and ventricles represent the electrical activity of the heart in an electrocardiogram (ECG). In addition to providing information about the heart's fundamental rhythms, an ECG also serves as an indicator for a variety of abnormalities. This includes abnormalities such as arrhythmia, a shortened QT interval, myocardial ischemia and other conditions. There have been numerous studies using IoT to monitor ECGs in the past research work. The IoT-founded ECG observing scheme projected in [20] consists of devices that receive data wirelessly. In order to perceive cardiac irregularities in actual time, it used an automated search method. It was proposed in [21] that an ECG monitoring system be integrated into a t-shirt. The ECG data was collected using a bio potential chip. Bluetooth was used to deliver the recorded data to the end users. A mobile app could be used to view the ECG data that had been recorded. 5.2 mW is the minimum amount of power required to run the proposed system. After integrating big data analytics into an IoT system, real-time monitoring can be achieved. Notably, the authors in [22] have attempted to address the problem of high power ingesting with a wearable ECG nursing scheme. Compressive sensing, a new method they've proposed, has the potential to reduce power consumption while also enhancing ECG monitoring performance. It has been reported that an IoT-founded drop recognition and ECG observing scheme using a bank of cloud founded server and a movable submission has been developed. Elderly patients can be monitored in real time using this system's ECG and accelerometer data, which are constantly checked.

10.7.2 Monitoring of Blood Glucose

Diabetes is a health condition characterized by persistently elevated blood glucose levels. In humans, it is one of the most prevalent diseases. Type-1 diabetes, type-2 diabetes and gestational diabetes are the three most common forms of the disease. But the most common method of identifying diabetes is "fingerpicking" followed by blood glucose analysis. Noninvasive, comfortable, convenient and safe blood glucose monitoring devices have benefited from recent advances in IoT technology. IPv6 connectivity was used to connect the wearable sensors to the healthcare providers. Researchers have developed a glove that uses a Raspberry Pi camera to measure blood glucose levels, as well as a visible laser beam. The diabetic condition of the patients was determined by analyzing a set of images taken from the fingertip. With IoT architecture, researchers were able to measure blood glucose levels using a double moving average algorithm [23].

10.7.3 Monitoring of Body Temperature

Many diagnostic procedures use the body temperature of a patient as an indicator of whether or not the patient is in a state of homeostasis. Certain sicknesses for example trauma, sepsis, and so on can cause changes in body temperature, which can be a warning sign. Many diseases require clinicians to make implications around the healthiness position of their patients by monitoring their temperature over time. However, the patient's discomfort and the high risk of infection are always a problem with these methods. This problem has been addressed in a number of ways by the recent advancements in IoT-based technologies. Infrared sensors embedded in the tympanic membrane of a 3D printed UWB localizer were projected in [24] for monitoring the body's core temperature. A wireless instrument module and a data dispensation component were built into the device. Fever is not influenced by the surrounding corporal action in this case. With the help of Arduino and Raspberry Pi, Gunawan has created an Internet of Things (IoT) temperature monitoring system. It was possible to access the temperature data via a desktop computer or a mobile phone, and the data was stored in a database. Other studies have used wearable and lightweight sensors to monitor infants' body temperatures in real time. It can also notify parents if the temperature rises above a certain threshold.

10.7.4 THE MEASUREMENT OF BLOOD PRESSURE

Blood pressure (BP) measurement is an essential part of any diagnostic procedure. A person must be present to record blood pressure using the most common method. With IoT and other detecting skill integrated, BP monitoring has been transformed. Wearable cuffless devices have been proposed in [25] that can portion systolic and diastolic body fluid pressure simultaneously. Documented data can be stored on the internet. In addition, the method's effectiveness and accuracy were both evaluated on a sample of 60 people. Guntha's IoT-based BP measurement system uses cloud computing and fog computing. A long-term real-time monitoring system was now in place after this step was taken. Documented information can also be saved on the device for future use. Deep learning-based CNN models were used to evaluate systolic and diastolic lifeblood force in additional training. In [26], an ECG signal and a photoplethysmogram (PPG) documented from the sensitized were projected for the measurement of blood pressure. The attached microcontroller module was used to calculate the BP, and the recorded data were then sent to the cloud storage.

10.7.5 BLOOD OXYGEN CONTENT MEASURING

An important parameter in healthcare analysis involves the use of pulse oximetry, which is a noninvasive way to measure oxygen saturation. The conventional approach has drawbacks, and the noninvasive method eliminates them while still allowing for real-time monitoring. The incorporation of IoT-founded skill into pulse oximetry has revealed prospective for use in the healthcare business. Body fluid oxygen inundation levels and heart degree and beat constraints could be measured using a noninvasive tissue oximeter that was proposed in [27]. A medicinal interference pronouncement was completed based on the recorded data. When oxygen saturation drops below a certain level, an alarm system is activated to notify the patient. The Blynk server was used to connect a pulse oximeter and a WLAN router to the system. A multispectral sensor proposed by Von Chong et al. reduces the negative impact of a solitary LED.

10.7.6 MONITORING OF ASTHMA

Asthma is a long-term condition that can cause breathing difficulties. Asthma causes the airways to swell, resulting in a narrowing of the passages. Breathlessness, coughing, ribcage discomfort and shortage of breath are all symptoms of this. An asthma attack can strike at any time, and the only thing that can save you is an inhaler or nebulizer. Real-time monitoring of this condition may be necessary. Recent years have seen an influx of IoT-based systems for asthma monitoring [28]. Asthma patients could benefit from a smart sensor-based HIoT solution that could monitor their respiratory rate. For diagnostic and monitoring purposes, the health data was stowed in a cloud server that was accessible to the caregivers. It was Raji's idea to use an LM35 hotness measuring device to monitor the breathing degree and send an alarm. Monitoring the hotness of the air breathed in and breathed out helped achieve this. The health center received and displayed the respiration data over the internet. Upon reaching a certain threshold, the patient was automatically alerted and a message was sent to their smartphone. Asthma patients were monitored and warned about their condition by the proposed system, which also advised them on the correct dosage of medication to take. In addition, the system was able to analyze the patient's environment and direct him or her out of a location that was detrimental to his or her well-being. Using IoT-based devices and machine knowledge, cloud calculating and big data investigation, it is possible to track asthma symptoms in real time. Researchers recommend a list of topographies that could be additional to the IoT-based asthma monitoring system in the future.

10.7.7   MOOD OBSERVATION AND TRACKING

Emotional health can be maintained by tracking one's mood, which can be used to monitor one's emotional well-being. Mental health professionals can also benefit from it, as it aids in the treatment of a wide range of mental illnesses. The ability to keep tabs on one's own emotional state is one of the many benefits of self-monitoring. A CNN net was applied to assess and classify a individual's temperament into six classes: pleased, enthusiastic, unhappy, peaceful, distraught and annoyed, rendering to temperament mining approach. An interactive system called "Meezaj" was used in a similar way to measure practical-time mood. Using the app, policymakers were able to identify the factors significant to the happiness in an educational institute. Now, thanks to an progressive machine knowledge procedure, heartbeat rate can be used to detect stress before it occurs. As an added benefit, patients' stress levels can be relayed to the system via communication. An IoT-based system that prevents an accident can be designed by analyzing the stress condition of a person. There are four negative emotions/moods that researchers have projected a wearable device can approximate. The intelligent system determines whether or not the driver is in a subconscious state by investigating the dissimilarity in these sentiments. The dc motor of the vehicle is stopped once the driver is in a trance-like state.

10.8   CONCLUSION

The HIoT scheme was examined in detail in this study. HIoT systems, their components, and how they communicate with one another have all been thoroughly examined in this document. This chapter also discusses the current state of healthcare services that are utilizing IoT-founded skills. As a result of using these concepts, IoT-technology has enabled healthcare professionals to monitor and diagnose a variety of health issues, measure a wide range of health parameters, and establish remote diagnostic facilities. As a result, healthcare has shifted from being centered around hospitals to being centered around patients. We've also talked about the HIoT systems various applications and recent trends. The HIoT system's design, manufacturing, and use have been described in detail, along with the challenges and issues they pose. Research and development in the next few years will be heavily influenced by these challenges. Furthermore, researchers who are keen to initiate their individual investigation and make aids to the arena of HIoT strategies will find complete info that is recent and up-to-date.

REFERENCES

[1] G. S. Pannu, M. D. Ansari, and P. Gupta, "Design and implementation of autonomous car using raspberry pi." International Journal of Computer Applications vol. 113, no. 9, 2015.

[2] V. N. Kumar, V. S. Reddy, and L. P. Sree, "design and development of accelerometer based system for driver safety." International Journal of Science, Engineering and Technology Research, vol. 3, p. 12, 2014.

[3] C. Hahn, S. Feld, and H. Schroter, "Predictive collision management for time and risk dependent path planning," in Proceedings of the 28th International Conference on Advances in Geographic Information Systems, ser. SIGSPATIAL '20. New York, NY, USA: Association for Computing Machinery, 2020, pp. 405–408.

[4] G. N. A. H. Yar, A.-B. Noor-ul Hassan, and H. Siddiqui, "Real-time shallow water image retrieval and enhancement for low-cost unmanned underwater vehicle using raspberry pi," in Proceedings of the 36th Annual ACM Symposium on Applied Computing, ser. SAC '21. New York, NY, USA: Association for Computing Machinery, 2021, pp. 1891–1899.

[5] V. G. Menon, "An IoT-enabled intelligent automobile system for smart cities," *Internet of Things*, pp. 100213, 2020.

[6] E. Qin, "Cloud computing and the internet of things: technology innovation in automobile service," in *Proceedings of the International Conference on Human Interface and the Management of Information*, pp. 173–180, Las Vegas, NV, USA, July 2013.

[7] I. Froiz-Míguez, T. Fernández-Caramés, P. Fraga-Lamas, and L. Castedo, "Design, implementation and practical evaluation of an IoT home automation system for fog computing applications based on MQTT and ZigBee-WiFi sensor nodes," *Sensors*, vol. 18, no. 8, p. 2660, 2018.

[8] P. S. Mathew, "Applications of IoT in healthcare," in *Cognitive Computing for Big Data Systems over IoT*, pp. 263–288, Springer, Berlin, Germany, 2018.

[9] V. Jagadeeswari, "A study on medical Internet of Things and Big Data in personalized healthcare system," *Health Information Science And Systems*, vol. 6, p. 14, 2018.

[10] H. Peng, Y. Tian, J. Kurths, L. Li, Y. Yang, and D. Wang, "Secure and energy-efficient data transmission system based on chaotic compressive sensing in body-to-body networks," *IEEE Transactions on Biomedical Circuits and Systems*, vol. 11, no. 3, pp. 558–573, 2017.

[11] A. Gatouillat, Y. Badr, B. Massot, and E. Sejdic, "Internet of medical things: a review of recent contributions dealing with cyber-physical systems in medicine," *IEEE Internet of Things Journal*, vol. 5, no. 5, pp. 3810–3822, 2018.

[12] L. M. Dang, M. J. Piran, D. Han, K. Min, and H. Moon, "A survey on internet of things and cloud computing for healthcare," *Electronics*, vol. 8, no. 7, p. 768, 2019.

[13] B. Oryema, "Design and implementation of an interoperable messaging system for IoT healthcare services," in *Proceedings of the 2017 14th IEEE Annual Consumer Communications & Networking Conference (CCNC)*, pp. 45–52, Las Vegas, NV, January 2017.

[14] A. Ahad, M. Tahir, and K.-L. A. Yau, "5G-based smart healthcare network: architecture, taxonomy, challenges and future research directions," *IEEE Access*, vol. 7, pp. 100747–100762, 2019.

[15] M. N. Birje and S. S. Hanji, "Internet of things based distributed healthcare systems: a review," *Journal of Data, Information and Management*, vol. 2, 2020.

[16] K. T. Kadhim, "An overview of patient's health status monitoring system based on internet of things (IoT)," *Wireless Personal Communications*, vol. 114, pp. 1–28, 2020.

[17] Y. Yuehong, "The internet of things in healthcare: an overview," *Journal of Industrial Information Integration*, vol. 1, pp. 3–13, 2016.

[18] G. Shanmugasundaram and G. Sankarikaarguzhali, "An investigation on IoT healthcare analytics," *International Journal of Information Engineering and Electronic Business*, vol. 9, no. 2, p. 11, 2017.

[19] J.-Y. Lee and R. A. Scholtz, "Ranging in a dense multipath environment using an UWB radio link," *IEEE Journal on Selected Areas in Communications*, vol. 20, pp. 1677–1683, 2002.

[20] H. Aftab, K. Gilani, J. Lee, L. Nkenyereye, S. Jeong, and J. Song, "Analysis of identifiers in IoT platforms," *Digital Communications and Networks*, vol. 6, no. 3, pp. 333–340, 2020.

[21] G. Cerruela García, I. Luque Ruiz, and M. Gómez-Nieto, "State of the art, trends and future of Bluetooth low energy, near field communication and visible light communication in the development of smart cities," *Sensors*, vol. 16, no. 11, p. 1968, 2016.

[22] R. Peng and M. L. Sichitiu, "Angle of arrival localization for wireless sensor networks," in *Proceedings of the 2006 3rd Annual IEEE Communications Society on Sensor and Ad Hoc Communications and Networks*, pp. 374–382, Reston, Virginia, September 2006.

[23] D. P. Young, "Ultra-wideband (UWB) transmitter location using time difference of arrival (TDOA) techniques," in *Proceedings of the Thirty-Seventh Asilomar Conference on Signals, Systems & Computers*, pp. 1225–1229, Pacific Grove, CA, USA, November 2003.

[24] R. Zetik, "UWB localization-active and passive approach [ultra wideband radar]," in *Proceedings of the 21st IEEE Instrumentation and Measurement Technology Conference (IEEE Cat. No. 04CH37510)*, pp. 1005–1009, Como, Italy, May 2004.

[25] R. J. Fontana and S. J. Gunderson, "Ultra-wideband precision asset location system," in *Proceedings of the 2002 IEEE Conference on Ultra Wideband Systems and Technologies (IEEE Cat. No. 02EX580)*, pp. 147–150, Baltimore, MD, USA, May 2002.

[26] L. Syed, S. Jabeen, M. S., and A. Alsaeedi, "Smart healthcare framework for ambient assisted living using IoMT and big data analytics techniques," *Future Generation Computer Systems*, vol. 101, pp. 136–151, 2019.

[27] G. Marques and R. Pitarma, "An indoor monitoring system for ambient assisted living based on internet of things architecture," *International Journal of Environmental Research and Public Health*, vol. 13, no. 11, p. 1152, 2016.

[28] A. Dohr, "The internet of things for ambient assisted living," in *Proceedings of the 2010 Seventh International Conference on Information Technology: New Generations*, pp. 804–809, Las Vegas, NA, USA, April 2010.

11 DDoS Attack Detection Using Predictive Machine Learning (ML) Algorithms in Wireless Body Area Network Environments

Bachu Taye Welteji,[1] Basant Tiwari,[1] Solomon D. Kebede,[1] Shailendra Gupta,[2] and Vivek Tiwari[3]
[1] Hawassa University Institute of Technology, Hawassa, Ethiopia
[2] Lakshmi Narain College of Technology, Bhopal, Madhya Pradesh, India
[3] Dr. S. P. Mukherjee IIIT-NR, Raipur, Chhattisgarh, India

CONTENTS

DOI: 10.1201/9781003145035-11

11.1   BACKGROUND

These days, technological advancements, mainly in micro-electromechanical systems (MEMS) and wireless communications are growing tremendously and becoming one of the leading forces to improve human living and lifestyle through combining sensor and communication technology. A wireless sensor network (WSN) is made up of a group of sensors nodes that communicate with one another via self-organized and multi-hop communication. A WSN is primarily used to monitor physical or biological conditions such as sound, temperature, pressure, and physiological variables, as well as to collaboratively convey sensed data over the network to a database server or physical recipient [1] [2].

Wireless body area networks (WBAN) is one of the sub fields of WSN. WBAN is a specialized WSN that has the potential to revolutionize healthcare monitoring. WBAN is composed of medical sensors equipped on a patient's body to sense the physiological values from the body. These values are communicated wirelessly with a gateway device, that is also installed with patients. These devices can be PDA, or any mobile phone, which can memorize, examine and communicate vital physiological values in real-time to a database server. These database servers can be installed either at the hospital site or any cloud-based platform. Wireless body area networks (WBANs) allow a patient to be free of the boundaries of a laboratory while yet allowing researchers and physicians to watch them. Without the use of intrusive video equipment, researchers can investigate disorders in real-world settings. Without increasing clinical visits, healthcare providers can acquire a larger understanding of a patient's health [3]. An example scenario of a WBAN medical application [4] is depicted in Figure 11.1.

Growth of the WBAN is getting higher and higher day by day, but with this higher usage, new techniques to attack on this technology are also growing. Thus, security in WBAN for healthcare applications is predominantly significant because sensitive physiological signs must be protected from unlawful usage for personal rewards and deceitful acts. Various cyberattacks are on the rise in today's internet era, putting the cybersecurity chain at risk. In the interest of cyber criminals, they want to manipulate individuals and hospitals to divulge important and sensitive data. For this purpose,

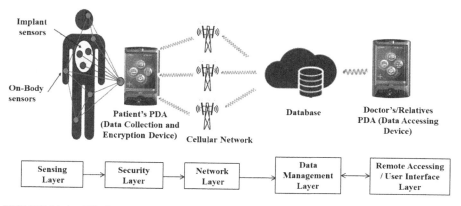

FIGURE 11.1 Wireless body area network (WBAN): medical application scenario.

hacking is a technological method of gaining access to a hospital's database servers and networks for harmful intentions, such as obtaining information to endanger a patient's life. As a result, WBAN has to be secure against these cyberattacks [5]. Thus, healthcare is more vulnerable to cyberattacks than other industries due to inherent security flaws. It is one of the most targeted industries in the world, with 81 percent of 223 healthcare organizations surveyed, and over 110 million patient records exposed in the United States alone in 2015 [6].

Among the most serious threats to the internet is DDoS attacks and they may do significant damage to communities, businesses and governments. With the emergence of new technologies, such as cloud computing, WSN, IoT, and artificial intelligence techniques, attackers can conduct DDoS attacks at a minimal cost, making them far more difficult to identify and block. In recent years, many IT-based companies have been affected by DDoS attacks. In 2020, however, DDoS attacks took on greater significance for healthcare providers as more hospitals than ever were targeted. Hackers use this attack to take down the servers, networks and applications by overloading them.

According to a Netscout analysis [7] on last year's threat landscape, cybercriminals increasingly preyed on the healthcare industry during the COVID-19 pandemic as firms transitioned to remote work and employed internet services for viral testing and immunizations. Malicious access requests and trash data submitted to healthcare systems increased in 2020, according to Cloudflare [8], an online infrastructure business.

To face such kind of attacks, organization and healthcare sectors are using various kinds of technological services including firewalls and intrusion detection/prevention system (IDS/IPS). An intrusion detection system (IDS) can be implemented as a software or hardware solution to detect intrusions and hazards, such as a DDoS attack, within an organization's ICT system. Signature or rule-based IDSs are distinguished from anomaly-based IDSs. The signature-based detection technique compares available facts to previously recorded and stored signatures in the IDS database. This method, however, can only detect known dangers and has a low rate of false alarms. In contrast to the first technique, an anomaly based intrusion detection system observes the behaviour of an event and finds any anomalies. As a result, it may detect an unidentified attack but with a greater false alarm rate [9]. The latest trend in detecting a DDoS attack is using data mining and/or machine learning (ML) techniques which are both fast and accurate in detecting a DDoS attack.

Data mining is defined as the method of mining or extracting information or knowledge from an enormous volume of data. In other words, it's used to extract knowledge/data from a large dataset. It is also used for finding relative patterns from a dataset [10]. Since, well-designed techniques of data mining are available, DDoS prevention has technologically advanced rapidly [10]. The huge volume of existing and afresh appearing network data influenced researchers to use data mining technologies for investigation of attacks since it requires more processing over voluminous data inside dataset [11]. Currently, data mining approaches have been frequently utilized and a number of researches are continuing for developing an effective IDS system, due to the fact that data mining methods are suitable for mining a wide range of benign and malicious traffic from a network flow. This can be very supportive for differentiating the incoming packets, so that such studies can effectively predict whether packets received are valid or not (i.e. an attack packet) [12].

Similarly, machine learning has developed as a powerful tool for system security, including authentication and verification, identity management, anti-jamming dumping, and malware discovery. Network and routing tasks, as well as network security, have all benefited from machine learning [13]. Data mining techniques are used to examine various attack patterns in the network. Many classifications, clustering, and classification via clustering (CvC) algorithms are available to analyze the data.

None of the existing detection and prevention mechanism of DDoS attacks are fully satisfactory to the IT world. That's why some of the giant IT companies are suffering by these attacks. According to [14], the biggest DDoS attack, i.e. flooding, took place in February, 2018. GitHub, a famous online code management service used by millions of developers, was the target of the attack. This attack peaked at 1.3 TBPS of inbound traffic and 126.9 million packets per second of outgoing traffic. In October of 2016, the second largest DDoS attack was launched on Dyn, a major DNS provider. Many big websites were affected by this attack, including AirBnB, Netflix, PayPal, Visa, Amazon, The New York Times, Reddit and GitHub.

This influenced the researcher to propose an effective machine learning technique that detects flooding types of DDoS. This work analyzed six machine learning algorithms including Adabost, Jrip, J48, k-NN, Random Committee and Random Forest for classification and detection of DDoS attack under KDD-NSL and latest CICIDS 2017 dataset to detect the attack packets by these classification techniques. Further, this study recommends the best classification algorithm for detection of DDoS attack. Finally, the study will give some directions as to future work as well.

These algorithms are implemented and evaluated individually with different types of datasets available to get accuracy of detection. The proposed study concludes the best available machine learning algorithm with taking old and newer datasets to detect the DDoS attack. This study focused on following major research questions:

- Which machine learning technique is better performed to detect the DDoS attack?
- Which dataset is best suitable to get accuracy of detection of DDoS attack?

11.2   WIRELESS BODY AREA NETWORK (WBAN)

Wireless body area network is group of sensor nodes fitted onto a patient's body for reading of physiological data and then sending it to remote devices like a database server or healthcare provider [15]. But this requires fulfilling some open challenges. For example, sensing devices should be small with limited battery resources so that they can be easily wearable. There should be an intermediate device that has a capability to send sensed data and must be portable and small so that it can be ported with patient body, so that whenever patient moves this device can also be moved.

11.2.1   WBAN Hardware Components

WBAN hardware encompasses a set of sensory nodes and gateway devices [16] (see Figure 11.2). WBAN hardware components are basically classified into three categories, these are:

- **Gateway/personal device**: gateway can be also called coordinator, aggregator or hub. It is a device which gathers physiological data received from the sensor nodes and actuators. Further, it can forward them to the user (e.g. the patient, a nurse, a doctor) or database server via an external gateway. Examples

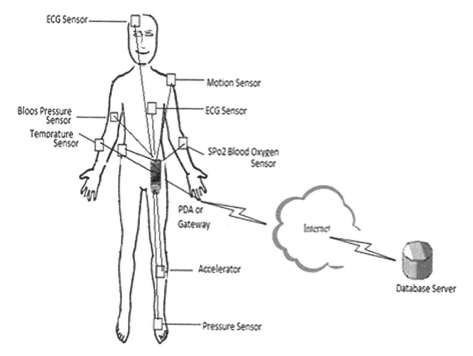

FIGURE 11.2   Wireless body area network with technological configuration.

of personal devices are laptop, personal digital assistant (PDA) and smart-phone [17].

- **Actuator**: this is a device that can execute activities based on data reported by sensor nodes or by interacting with users. For example, based on glucose level monitoring, an actuator with a reservoir and an integrated pump can deliver the precise dose of insulin to diabetic patients.
- **Sensor nodes**: these are the medical sensors which sense the actual physiological data from the patient's body and send them to the personal device or PDA. Actuators can be integrated with the sensor. There are various types of biomedical sensor nodes available in the market for healthcare applications including accelerometer, CO_2 gas, blood glucose, blood oxygen, EEG, ECG, temperature, etc. [17].

11.2.2 Communication Model for WBAN

The communication model of WBAN is generally categorized into three levels that are intra-WBAN, inter-WBAN and beyond-WBAN communication at different tiers [18]. Figure 11.3 illustrates the high-level communication model of a WBAN system. As the figure shows, biomedical sensors, such as electroencephalograph (EEG), electrocardiograph (ECG), electromyography (EMG) or blood pressure measuring sensors are positioned on the human body to gather physiological values of a patient's

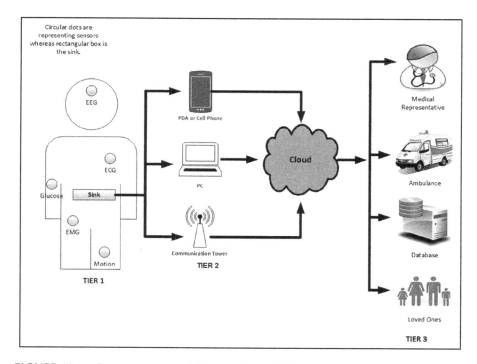

FIGURE 11.3   Communication architecture of a WBAN.

body [19]. These are arranged at tier-1. The data assembled from these sensors are then forwarded to the coordinator or sink node (e.g. smartphone, PDA). The sink at tier-1 transmits the collected data to the next communication level through an access point (AP). The tier-3 of communication involves a healthcare provider, like medical doctor or a medical center or any medical data repository which receives sensed data from AP.

11.3 MACHINE LEARNING IN DDOS ATTACK DETECTION

Machine learning is a technology that allows automated systems to be built. These systems can also learn from previous experiences and examine historical data. It gives results based on its previous experience. ML is concerned with categorization and prediction based on previously learnt attributes from the training data [20]. A domain goal (problem formulation) is required for ML algorithms (e.g. dependent variable to predict). Nowadays, ML is widely utilized to detect the attack which contains malicious data and packet over the network including DDoS attack.

11.3.1 TYPES OF MACHINE LEARNING ALGORITHMS

Depending on their purpose machine learning algorithms can be divided into various categories including classification or supervised, clustering or unsupervised, semi-supervised and reinforcement learning. This research employed classification or supervised learning methods, which entail a two-step procedure that includes both learning and classification. The learning step creates the classification model, and the classification step categorizes the data, with the model predicting class labels for supplied data [21]. In this category, 59 algorithms are available in WEKA 3.9.2 by different classifier technique (like Bayes, Lazy, Rules, Tree, etc.) [22]. This study utilized six classification algorithms that are named as follows:

1. k-nearest-neighbor classifiers
2. Decision tree
3. JRIP algorithm
4. AdaBoost algorithm
5. Random forest algorithm
6. Random committee algorithm

These algorithms are utilized for classification and detection of DDoS attack. These algorithms are implemented and evaluated individually to get accuracy of detection. The study uses NSL-KDD dataset and latest dataset CICIDS2017, dedicated for DDoS attack [29].

11.4 RELATED WORK

Many researchers have proposed various detection strategies for identifying the cyber threat caused by DDoS attacks. Among those studies, this section will highlight several related works aimed at improving DDoS attack detection.

In [23] the authors discussed an assessment of data mining-based Fuzzy C-Means clustering and K-Means clustering algorithms by using NSL-KDD repository for recognizing the classification of the significant attacks, i.e. DoS, Root-to-Local, User-to-Root and probing attack. Fuzzy C-Means clustering algorithm detects 45.95% attacks and K-Means algorithm detects 44.72% attacks on NSL-KDD dataset with 28 attributes. Other classification algorithms like SVM, Naive Bayesian Networks and AdaBoost are the algorithms used by [24]. Author used core vector machines (CVM) as the classifier used for data mining. It gives them somehow ideal execution. It identified an attack in a wide range with a worthy discovery percentage and bogus positive rate. It required some investment for preparing tests contrasted with different classifiers like SVM. For every kind of violence, a CVM model is built and then their outcomes are joined using a weighted function. This model claimed about 99% discovery percentage and 27% bogus positive percentage. In [25], the author discussed a semi-supervised machine learning way to deal with DDoS attacks classification. It began from an unlabeled traffic measurement acquired against three attributes for target guard (for example, web server is an example for victim/target). The attributes incorporated, CPU usage, traffic rate and processing delay. The two distinctive clustering technique and voting technique can be chosen for the naming of the traffic stream for the unlabeled data. The tuples falling in inverse groups are named with an extra class called 'Suspicious'. RF, KNN and SVM classification technique like RF, SVM and k-NN are applied on classified data to group DDoS attacks. The test consequences of 96.66%, 95% and 92% honesty scores were accomplished with RF, KNN and SVM models correspondingly under improved parameter adjustments inside given arrangements of values. By using descriptive subdivision of CICIDS2017 dataset with latest attack types, the method was additionally approved for the precision of label assignments. It appeared to be encouraging as they acquire over 82% correct labels.

The author in [26] presented new techniques to defend against a set of active attacks, like DoS, probe, vampire and U2R in MANET. The author offered behaviour-based and distributed trust-based analysis under the AODV routing protocol in NS-2. The author in [27] used the feed-forward back propagation method as a classifier to handle MANET against DDoS attacks under AODV protocol. Authors claimed improvement in PDR and throughput and a significant reduction in delay. The author in [28] presented a rate-limiting scheme to protect the network against DDoS attacks. It immediately eliminates that node from the network as found the attacker node.

11.5   MATERIAL AND METHODS

This section focusses on research methods and study design used, and approach of data collection, management and analysis.

11.5.1   DATASET

There are so many databases available which are widely accessible and used for the DDoS related research. Some of them are: FIFA World Cup Dataset 1998, KDD99 and NSL-KDD, DARPA 2009, CAIDA, DEFCON, UNSW-NB15, CICIDS2017.

But, most of the datasets are outdated. The analysis of DDoS attack in this study is done by using two different datasets. The first one is CICISD2017 and the second one is NSL-KDD datasets.

11.5.2 DESCRIPTION OF THE DATASET

The CICIDS2017 dataset [29] was designed to fill in the gaps in the previous datasets. Because intrusion attack types evolve and become more complex, a prevalent issue is obsolete data, which affects the majority of datasets. A lack of features and metadata, as well as a lack of variety in known threats, have been highlighted in several datasets. A complete and well-rounded methodology for developing IDS/IPS benchmarking dataset is necessary, according to the authors. Unsupervised datamining approaches, such as classification algorithms, require labeled data sets for training [30]. Furthermore, the authors stress the importance of having a perfect data set: the ideal network-based data set is current, properly labeled, publicly available and includes real network traffic, including all forms of attacks and typical user behaviour, as well as payload, over a long period of time. These conditions are met by the CICIDS2017 dataset [31]. CICIDS2017 is the most up-to-date dataset when compared to other datasets, as it includes the most recent attack types such as DoS, DDoS, brute force SSH, brute force FTP, Heartbleed, penetration and botnet [29].

This research is focused on DDoS attack dataset. It has 225,745 records and 79 attributes including the label/class attribute. The label attribute has two distinct values, i.e. Benign and DDoS. Benign has 97718 records and DDoS has 128,027 records. Figure 11.4 shows the DDoS dataset label distribution in CICIDS 2017 dataset.

This work also uses NSL-KDD dataset for DDoS attack. It has 223,112 records and 42 attributes including the label/class attribute. The label attribute has two distinct values, i.e. Benign and DDoS. Benign has 95,096 records and DDoS has 128,016 records. Figure 11.5 shows the DDoS dataset label distribution in NSL-KDD dataset [32].

11.5.3 DATASET PRE-PROCESSING

The majority of existing datasets have unwanted features that includes missing or redundant values that must be removed during pre-processing.

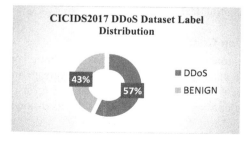

FIGURE 11.4 CICIDS2017-DDoS dataset features distribution.

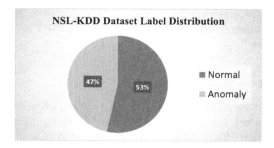

FIGURE 11.5   NSL-KDD dataset features distribution.

11.5.4   DATASET CLEANING

Before starting to use any dataset, cleaning the dataset is mandatory. The researcher makes sure about the neatness of the data and it is directly related to the output of the research. Thus, it is mandatory to clean the nominated CICIDS 2017 dataset from errors. Removing the redundant attribute '**Fwd_Header_Length**' that appeared twice and "**Destination_port**" attribute also removed because it is used only for specific machine. The total number of attributes become 77. The dataset cannot load to the WEKA if you have a redundant attribute name.

Furthermore, redundant 2633 data out of 225,745 records have been also dropped and 223,112 records remain in the dataset. There were two attributes that had missing values:

1.   In 'Total Length of Bwd packet' attribute four missing values and
2.   In 'Flow Bytes/s' one missing value.

All missing values for nominal and numeric properties in a dataset are replaced with the training data's modes and means. By default, the class attribute is ignored. This is all done by '**Replace MissingValues**' algorithm in WEKA [22].

11.5.5   FEATURES SELECTION

The feature selection is accomplished in this study using filtering approach. In the filtering method there are a lot of algorithms. This study follows information gain and gain ratio attribute selection techniques.

11.5.5.1   Information Gain

If the presence of a feature and the matching class distribution are available, information gain (IG) estimates the totality of information in bits about the class prediction. It expresses the projected entropy reduction in concrete terms. Thus, it is needed to calculate two kinds of entropy using frequency tables as follows:

1.   Entropy based on one attribute's frequency table:
     i.e. calculate entropy of the target/parent.

$$E(T) = \sum_{i=1}^{k} - pi \, log2 \, pi \qquad (1)$$

Where pi signifies the amount of instances belonging to class i ($i = 1, \ldots, k$).

2. Entropy based on two characteristics' frequency tables:
    i.e. the dataset is fragmented on the different attributes. The entropy for each division is calculated. Further, it is added proportionately to find total entropy of the split.

$$E(T,X) = \sum_{c \in X} P(c) E(c) \qquad (2)$$

Where T denotes parent class, X denotes parent attribute, $P(c)$ attribute value and $E(c)$ entropy of attribute value.

The resulting entropy found by equation two is deducted from the entropy earlier split, i.e. from equation one. The result is the information gain.

$$Gain(T,X) = Entropy(T) - Entropy(T,X) \qquad (3)$$

Where Entropy(T) denotes parent entropy, i.e. entropy of class attribute, and Entropy(T, X) denotes entropy of single attribute, i.e. equation two.

11.5.5.2　Gain Ratio

The gain ratio is a bias-reducing variation of the information gain. It is used to lessen the bias towards multi-valued features by taking into account the number and size of branches when selecting an attribute. The intrinsic information is represented by the entropy of the distribution of instances into branches. That's how much data we'll need to figure out which branch a given instance belongs to. The value of an attribute decreases as intrinsic information increases.

The split information value signifies the potential information produced by dividing the training dataset D into v splits, equivalent to v outcomes on attribute A.

$$SplitInfo_A(D) = -\sum_{j=1}^{v} \frac{|D_j|}{|D|} \times log_2 \left(\frac{|D_j|}{[D]} \right) \qquad (4)$$

The gain ratio is defined as:

$$GainRatio(Attribute) = \frac{Gain(Attribute)}{Intrinsic\_info(Attribute)} \qquad (5)$$

By applying feature selection method with ranking algorithm, the output of the dataset attributes are ranked. According to the algorithm, by taking the intersection

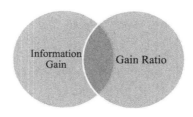

FIGURE 11.6   Intersection of information gain and gain ratio algorithms.

TABLE 11.1
Dataset Description before and after Pre-Processing

Dataset Name	Status	No. of records	No. of attributes	Size (MB)	DDoS	BENIGN
CICIDS-2017	Before	225,745	79	73.5	128,027	97,718
	After	223,112	67	64.1	128,016	95,096
NSL-KDD		125,973	42	17.8	58,630	67,343

of the two algorithms the irrelevant features are removed from the dataset. In both algorithms, 10 attributes are ranked 0 (zero). Figure 11.6 shows the intersection of IG and GR.

InfoGainAttributeEval ∩ GainRatioAttributeEval

Dataset after and before pre-processing is shown in Table 11.1.

11.6   WORKING ENVIRONMENT

In this sub section, we discuss the test bed for detection of DDoS attack.

11.6.1   Test Bed for Detection of a DDoS Attack

11.6.1.1   Software

WEKA 3.9.2 is the software program used to identify DDoS attacks. It was proposed in 1997 at the University of Waikato in New Zealand as a platform tool for data mining and machine learning activities. WEKA is a collection of data mining and machine learning algorithms [22].

11.6.1.2   Hardware

For the proposed work, we used Windows 10 Pro operating system with two GHz Intel processor with two cores and four logical processor. 16 GB RAM is utilized within the system and system type belong to x64-based PC.

Predicted class

		yes	no	Total
Actual class	yes	TP	FN	P
	no	FP	TN	N
	Total	P'	N'	P + N

FIGURE 11.7 Confusion matrix with total tuples including positive and negative.

11.6.2 Performance Metrics for Evaluating Classifiers

To determine how well a classifier predicts tuple class labels, performance metrics are utilized. Before understanding the performance metrics, we must know four building block concepts used in measuring the performance.

1. **True positives (TP)**: these are the positive tuples that the classifier successfully labeled.
2. **True negatives (TN)**: these are the negative tuples that the classifier correctly identified.
3. **False positives (FP)**: these are negative tuples that have been mistakenly categorized as positive.
4. **False negatives (FN)**: these are positive tuples that have been incorrectly categorized as negative.

The confusion matrix in Figure 11.7 summarizes the above phrases. The confusion matrix is a handy tool for determining how well a classifier recognizes tuples from various classes. TP and TN indicate when the classifier is correct, while FP and FN indicate when the classifier is incorrect (i.e. mislabeling).

- **Accuracy**: the percentage of test set tuples properly classified by a classifier on a given test set is referred to as accuracy of detection of classifier. That is,

$$\text{Accuracy} = \frac{TP + TN}{P + N} \quad (1)$$

- This is also known as the classifier's overall accuracy rate in most literature, and it refers to how well the classifier detects tuples from different classes. In the case of comparison, if the accuracy of one classifier is better that the others, it does not mean that this classifier is the best. There are other evaluation measures to be considered depending on the system.
- **Error rate**: it is also known as a classifier's misclassification rate, which is simply 1 − accuracy of classifier. It is calculated as:

$$\text{Error Rate} = \frac{FP + FN}{P + N} \quad (2)$$

- **Sensitivity**: the true positive (recognition) rate is another name for it (i.e. the number of positive tuples that are correctly recognized). It is calculated as:

$$\text{Sensitivity} = \frac{TP}{P} \tag{3}$$

- **Specificity**: it is a genuine negative rate (i.e. the quantity of negative tuples that are correctly acknowledged). This can be defined as:

$$\text{Specificity} = \frac{TN}{N} \tag{4}$$

- **Precision**: it can be thought of as a metric of exactness, i.e. how many of the tuples tagged as positive are actually positive? That is:

$$\text{Precision} = \frac{TP}{TP + FP} \tag{5}$$

- **Recall**: it is a metric of completeness, i.e. how many positive tuples are tagged as such? This can be calculated as:

$$\text{Recall} = \frac{TP}{P} \tag{6}$$

- **Speed**: this refers to the computation time and effort required to create and use the provided classifier for a given dataset.

11.6.3   Holdout Method and Random Sub Sampling

The dataset is divided into two distinct subsets, referred to as the training and testing datasets. The dataset is separated into a 66.6 percent training set and a 33.3 percent testing set for this investigation. Furthermore, the model is developed using the training set, while the model's accuracy is estimated using the test set. The estimate is pessimistic because just a part of the initial data was used to develop the model.

The holdout method is repeated k times in random subsampling, which is a version of the holdout method. The average of the accuracies gained from each iteration is used to calculate the overall accuracy estimate. The dataset split and the process of assessing accuracy is shown in Figure 11.8.

11.6.4   Cross-Validation

In k-fold cross-validation, the whole dataset is divided into totally unrelated k parts, based on the value of k, i.e. $X1, X2, \ldots, X_k$, and each subset is nearly of same data size.

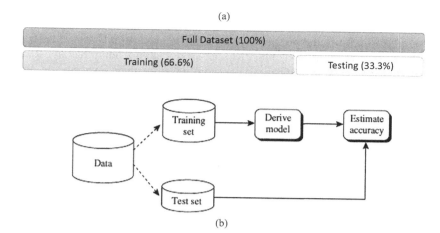

FIGURE 11.8 (a) Training and testing a data sample with the holdout method. (b) Assessing accuracy with the holdout method.

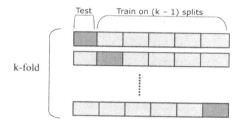

FIGURE 11.9 K-fold cross validation.

Model training is done by the total of k − 1 subset and the evaluation is done by the rest of the subset from the partitioned dataset. Both training and testing is going up to kth cycle. For the first round, the total of X2 up to X_k is used as training datasets and X1 used as model evaluation. For the second round, the total of X1, X3, X4, …, X_k is used as training dataset and X2 used as model evaluation or test set and the iteration will continue until k times as shown Figure 11.9. The accuracy of the classifier is calculated as:

$$\frac{\text{The sum of accurate classification from k round}}{\text{Entire tuples of the original data dataset}}$$

Finally, we may have more computational power to use more folds, but 10-fold cross-validation is suggested for evaluating accuracy, because of its comparatively low pre-conceived notion and variant.

11.7   PROPOSED ALGORITHM

In proposed algorithm, the pre-processed dataset is given to different classification algorithms, namely, AdaBoost, J48, JRip, KNN, Random Committee and Random Forest. That individual classification algorithm develops their own models. For all algorithms, the dataset, the experimental environment (like minimum and maximum memory allocation) and testing option is the same, individual algorithm evaluating the performance based on performance metrics. Based on the outcome of the evaluation, the comparison is done. Finally, the best classifier is selected for the classification of DDoS attack and Benign packet.

Proposed detection/classification DDoS attack from legitimate using AdaBoost, J48, JRip, KNN, Random Committee and Random Forest classification algorithms is shown as follows:

The proposed algorithm has the following steps that are also represented as a flow diagram shown in Figure 11.10.

1. Input dataset D1, D2.
2. Pre-process the dataset:
    a. replace missing values
    b. remove redundant values
    c. feature selection.

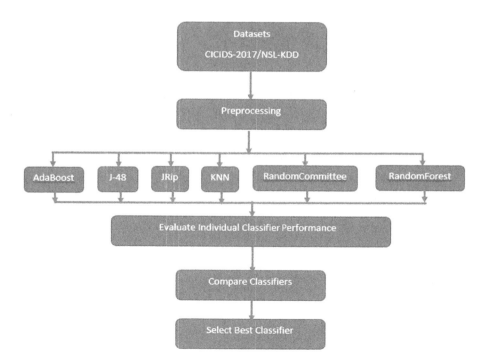

FIGURE 11.10   Model selection of classification method.

3. Apply AdaBoost algorithm on the pre-processed dataset:
   a. observe and analyse the performance.
4. Apply J-48 algorithm on the pre-processed dataset:
   a. observe and analyse the performance.
5. Apply JRip algorithm on the pre-processed dataset:
   a. observe and analyse the performance.
6. Apply KNN algorithm on the pre-processed dataset:
   a. observe and analyse the performance.
7. Apply Random Committee algorithm on the pre-processed dataset:
   a. observe and analyse the performance.
8. Apply Random Forest algorithm on the pre-processed dataset:
   a. observe and analyse the performance.
9. Compare evaluation performance of Step 3, 4, 5, 6, 7, 8.
10. Take the best classification based on evaluation performance from Step 9 and use as a classifier.

11.8   RESULTS AND DISCUSSION

The design and experimentation of selected algorithms with the major activities during the experiment are discussed in this section. The section also presents the achieved results with challenge and difficulties.

The detection process is started from dataset pre-processing up to final evaluation performance of individual algorithm.

11.8.1   RESULTS OF FEATURE SELECTION

In the dataset pre-processing, feature selection or attribute evaluation is one of steps. Depending on the result of the algorithms, the irrelevant attributes are removed and the dataset becomes more precise and lightweight. InfoGain AttributeEval and Gain RatioAttributeEval with ranker algorithm are used to select best features. Figures 11.11 and 11.12 show the output of both of the algorithms.

In both cases ten attributes are selected (i.e. attribute number 32, 33, 34, 50, 56, 57, 58, 59, 60 and 61) as irrelevant or ranked 0. That means ranked 0 attributes doesn't have any influence on the performance of the dataset.

11.8.2   CONFUSION MATRIX RESULT ON INDIVIDUAL ALGORITHMS

In this step, experimental performance evaluation of an individual algorithm is done on the pre-processed dataset. The algorithm performance is measured by using the same test option i.e. k-fold cross-validation, where k = 10. Tables 11.2 and 11.3 show the results obtained for confusion matrix for each selected algorithm over CICIDS 2017 dataset and NSL-KDD respectively.

11.8.3   RESULTS OF EVALUATION METRICS

In this subsection, performance metrics results for individual algorithm have been shown for CICIDS-2017 and NSL-KDD dataset in Tables 11.4 and 11.5 respectively.

```
0.002481     44  FIN Flag Count
0.000144     46  RST Flag Count
0.000144     51  ECE Flag Count
0            57  Fwd Avg Packets/Bulk
0            33  Fwd URG Flags
0            50  CWE Flag Count
0            56  Fwd Avg Bytes/Bulk
0            32  Bwd PSH Flags
0            34  Bwd URG Flags
0            61  Bwd Avg Bulk Rate
0            60  Bwd Avg Packets/Bulk
0            59  Bwd Avg Bytes/Bulk
0            58  Fwd Avg Bulk Rate

Selected attributes: 5,63,53,6,65,55,13,35,1,11,66,
                     54,9,7,36,24,21,22,62,3,67,68,
                     23,41,42,43,10,29,26,14,38,27,
                     4,64,40,37,12,28,18,15,19,2,16,
                     17,30,73,70,25,72,8,39,52,49,69,
                     20,76,74,47,77,31,45,75,71,48,44,
                     46,51,57,33,50,56,32,34,61,60,59,58 : 77
```

FIGURE 11.11   The output of information gain attribute evaluation with a ranker algorithm.

```
0.01778      77  Idle Min
0.00679      48  ACK Flag Count
0            34  Bwd URG Flags
0            58  Fwd Avg Bulk Rate
0            32  Bwd PSH Flags
0            50  CWE Flag Count
0            56  Fwd Avg Bytes/Bulk
0            59  Bwd Avg Bytes/Bulk
0            60  Bwd Avg Packets/Bulk
0            61  Bwd Avg Bulk Rate
0            57  Fwd Avg Packets/Bulk
0            33  Fwd URG Flags

Selected attributes: 1,7,65,6,12,54,9,49,55,13,67,66,63,
                     5,69,11,10,14,53,68,35,36,62,3,31,
                     45,41,40,71,64,4,8,29,26,27,39,43,
                     42,28,22,52,24,23,21,70,73,38,72,
                     44,46,51,30,37,18,2,25,19,75,15,47,
                     16,17,20,76,74,77,48,34,58,32,50,
                     56,59,60,61,57,33 : 77
```

FIGURE 11.12   The output of gain ratio attribute evaluation with a ranker algorithm.

The graph shown in Figure 11.13 summarizes the above results in a graphical way. The graph shown in Figure 11.14 summarizes the above results in a graphical way.

Figure 11.15 shows the performance analysis of individual algorithms based on model building time for the CICIDS-2017 dataset as well as the NSL-KDD dataset.

TABLE 11.2
Results of Confusion Matrix Generated from CICIDS-2017 Dataset for Various Algorithms after Dataset Pre-Processing

Algorithm	Actual Class	Predicted Class		Total
		BENIGN	Malicious	
AdaBoost	BENIGN	94,803	293	95,096
	Malicious	174	1,27,842	1,28,016
	Total	94,977	1,28,135	2,23,112
J48	BENIGN	95,080	16	95,096
	Malicious	15	128001	1,28,016
	Total	95,095	1,28,017	2,23,112
k-NN	BENIGN	95,030	66	95,096
	Malicious	27	1,27,989	1,28,016
	Total	95,057	1,28,055	2,23,112
JRip	BENIGN	95,076	20	95,096
	Malicious	17	1,27,999	1,28,016
	Total	95,093	1,28,019	2,23,112
Random Committee	BENIGN	95,083	13	95,096
	Malicious	29	1,27,987	1,28,016
	Total	95,112	1,28,000	2,23,112
Random Forest	BENIGN	95,089	7	95,096
	Malicious	29	1,27,987	1,28,016
	Total	95,118	1,27,994	2,23,112

11.8.4 RESULTS DISCUSSION ON DDoS ATTACK DETECTION

In this subsection, the experimental results on DDoS attack detection are discussed with challenges and difficulties.

For this experiment CICIDS-2017 and NSL-KDD dataset has been used. After pre-processing the dataset, the selected algorithms were evaluated. Pre-processing the dataset is directly related to the model building time of the algorithms.

In CICIDS-2017 dataset, detection accuracy, error rate, sensitivity, specificity, precision and model building time are the evaluation measures for six classifiers: AdaBoost, J48, k-NN, JRip, Random Committee and Random Forest.

TABLE 11.3

Results of Confusion Matrix Generated from NSL-KDD Dataset for Various Algorithms after Dataset Pre-Processing

		Predicted Class		
Algorithm	Actual Class	BENIGN	Malicious	Total
AdaBoost	BENIGN	64,639	2,704	67,343
	Malicious	4,219	54,411	58,630
	Total	68,858	57,115	1,25,973
J48	BENIGN	67,200	143	67,343
	Malicious	132	58,498	58,630
	Total	67,332	58,641	1,25,973
k-NN	BENIGN	67,189	154	67,343
	Malicious	167	58,463	58,630
	Total	67,356	58,617	1,25,973
JRip	BENIGN	67,252	91	67,343
	Malicious	156	58,474	58,630
	Total	67,408	58,565	1,25,973
Random Committee	BENIGN	67,313	30	67,343
	Malicious	83	58,547	58,630
	Total	67,396	58,577	1,25,973
Random Forest	BENIGN	67,319	24	67,343
	Malicious	80	58,550	58,630
	Total	67,399	58,574	1,25,973

By interpreting the results shown in Figure 11.12 shows that AdaBoost, J48, k-NN, JRip, Random Committee and Random Forest classifiers achieved 99.79%, 99.986%, 99.958%, 99.983%, 99.981% and 99.983% accuracy respectively. Based on the accuracy result, J-48 algorithm is more accurate algorithm for CICIDS-2017 dataset.

The other parameter is model building time for all classifiers takes 99.84, 49.05, 0.23, 208.34, 51.41 and 296.73 (respectively) seconds to build their model. Therefore, k-NN finished the model building in 0.23 seconds, but the accuracy is 99.95%, that is lower than J48. On the other hand, J48 algorithm takes 49.05 seconds to build the model and 99.985% accurate.

In NSL-KDD dataset, the accuracy of AdaBoost, J48, k-NN, JRip, Random Committee and Random Forest are 94.5%, 99.78%, 99.74%, 99.8% 99.91%, and

TABLE 11.4
Results of Algorithm Evaluation on CICIDS-2017 Dataset

Algorithm	Accuracy	Error rate	Sensitivity	Specificity	Precision	Model Building Time (sec)
AdaBoost	99.7906	0.2093	99.6918	99.864	99.8167	99.84
J48	99.9861	0.0139	99.9831	99.9882	99.9842	49.05
k-NN	99.9583	0.0417	99.9305	99.9789	99.9715	0.23
JRip	99.9834	0.0165	99.9789	99.9867	99.9821	208.34
Random Committee	99.9811	0.0188	99.9863	99.9773	99.9695	51.41
Random Forest	99.9838	0.0161	99.9926	99.9773	99.9695	296.73

TABLE 11.5
Results of Algorithm Evaluation on NSL-KDD Dataset

Algorithm	Accuracy (%)	Error rate (%)	Sensitivity (%)	Specificity (%)	Precision (%)	Model Building Time (sec)
AdaBoost	94.5043	5.4956	95.9847	92.804	93.8728	24.09
J48	99.7816	0.2183	99.7876	99.7748	99.8039	38.56
k-NN	99.7451	0.2548	99.7713	99.7151	99.752	0.03
JRip	99.8039	0.196	99.8648	99.7339	99.7685	182.12
Random Committee	99.9102	0.0897	99.9554	99.8584	99.9768	17.59
Random Forest	99.9174	0.0825	99.9808	99.8635	99.9362	110.67

99.917% respectively. For NSL-KDD dataset, Random Forest algorithm scored a higher accuracy than the other classifiers.

Model building time for AdaBoost, J48, k-NN, JRip, Random Committee and Random Forest are 24.09, 38.56, 0.03, 182.12, 17.59 and 110.67 seconds respectively. K-NN takes less time than the other in model building time. Model building time of each algorithm based on NSL-KDD dataset is lower than the CICIDS-2017

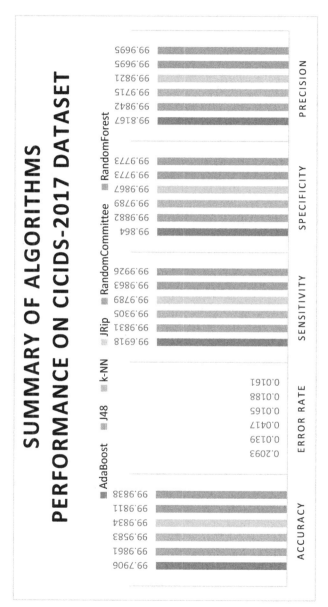

FIGURE 11.13   Algorithm performance evaluation on CICIDS-2017 dataset.

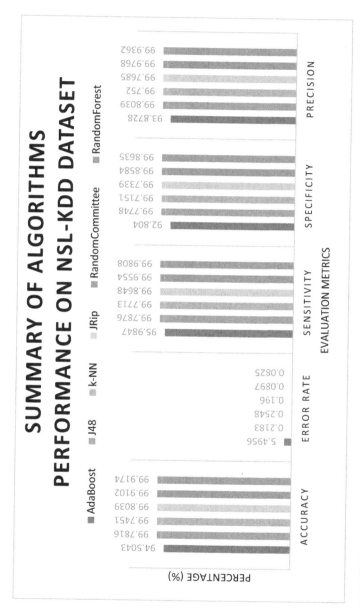

FIGURE 11.14 Algorithm performance evaluation on NSL-KDD dataset.

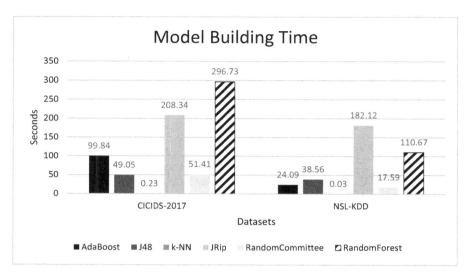

FIGURE 11.15   Performance analysis based on model building time.

dataset, because the number of instances in NSL-KDD dataset is lower than CICIDS-2017 dataset.

The main challenge was in testing of the dataset. Because of the enormousness of the dataset testing in k-fold is much more difficult. Especially in the case of JRip and k-NN. To overcome this challenge, the researcher tries to change the testing option but it has significant differences in the detection accuracy.

Finally, the researcher noticed that, the accuracy of the algorithm may or may not depend on the number of instances. For example, the accuracy of k-NN algorithm is the same before and after pre-processing (reducing) the dataset. But in the case of JRip and J48, there are some variations.

11.9   CONCLUSION

Wireless body area networks (WBANs) are one of the key technologies that support the development of pervasive health monitoring (remote patient monitoring systems), which has attracted more attention in recent years. These WBAN applications requires stringent security requirements as they are concerned with human lives. In the recent scenario of the corona pandemic, where most of the healthcare providers are giving online services for treatment, DDoS attacks become the major threats over the internet. This chapter particularly focusses on detection of DDoS attack using machine learning algorithm over healthcare environment. In the process of attack detection, the dataset is pre-processed. After pre-processing the dataset, the cleaned dataset is given to the popular classification algorithms in the area of machine learning namely, AdaBoost, J48, k-NN, JRip, Random Committee and Random Forest classifiers. Those algorithms are evaluated independently and the results are recorded. Result concluded that J48 outperform with accuracy of 99.98% with CICIDS dataset and Random Forest outperform with accuracy of 99.917%, but it takes longest model building time. Depending on the evaluation performance the appropriate classifier is selected for further DDoS detection at real-time.

REFERENCES

[1] Yick, J., Mukherjee, B., & Ghosal, D. (2008). Wireless sensor network survey. *Computer networks*, vol. 52, no. 12, pp. 2292–2330.

[2] Ko, J., Lu, C., Srivastava, M. B., Stankovic, J. A., Terzis, A., & Welsh, M. (2010). Wireless sensor networks for healthcare. *Proceedings of the IEEE*, 98(11), 1947–1960. *Proc.*

[3] Khan, R. A., & Pathan, A. S. K. (2018). The state-of-the-art wireless body area sensor networks: A survey. *International Journal of Distributed Sensor Networks*, *14*(4), 1550147718768994.

[4] Chakraborty, C., Gupta, B., & Ghosh, S. K. (2013). A review on telemedicine-based WBAN framework for patient monitoring. *Telemedicine and e-Health*, *19*(8), 619–626.

[5] Fan, K., Jiang, W., Li, H., & Yang, Y. (2018). Lightweight RFID protocol for medical privacy protection in IoT. IEEE Transactions on Industrial Informatics, 14(4), 1656–1665.

[6] Huang, H., Gong, T., Ye, N., Wang, R., & Dou, Y. (2017). Private and secured medical data transmission and analysis for wireless sensing healthcare system. IEEE Transactions on Industrial Informatics, 13(3), 1227–1237.

[7] Netscout. Latest NETSCOUT Threat Intelligence Report Highlights Unprecedented DDoS Attack Activity. www.netscout.com/threatreport, downloaded at 01/10/2021.

[8] Cloudflare. DDoS attack trends for 2021. https://blog.cloudflare.com/ddos-attack-trends-for-2021-q2/ downloaded on 01/10/2021.

[9] Prakash, A., Satish, M., Bhargav, T. S. S., & Bhalaji, N. (2016). Detection and mitigation of denial of service attacks using stratified architecture. *Procedia Computer Science*, *87*, 275–280.

[10] Yusof, M. A. M., Ali, F. H. M., & Darus, M. Y. (2017, November). Detection and defense algorithms of different types of DDoS attacks using machine learning. In *International Conference on Computational Science and Technology,* vol. 481, pp. 370–379.

[11] Luo, H., Chen, Z., Li, J., & Vasilakos, A. V. (2017). Preventing distributed denial-of-service flooding attacks with dynamic path identifiers. *IEEE Transactions on Information Forensics and Security*, *12*(8), 1801–1815.

[12] Proano, A., & Lazos, L. (2011). Packet-hiding methods for preventing selective jamming attacks. *IEEE Transactions on dependable and secure computing*, *9*(1), 101–114.

[13] Alzahrani, S., & Hong, L. (2018). Generation of DDoS attack dataset for effective IDS development and evaluation. *Journal of Information Security*, *9*(04), 225.

[14] The largest DDoS attacks of all time. www.cloudflare.com/learning/ddos /famous-ddos-attacks/ downloaded.

[15] Tiwari, B., & Kumar, A. (2015). Standard deviation (SD)-based data filtering technique for body sensor network data. *International Journal of Data Science*, *1*(2), 189–203.

[16] Tiwari, Basant, & Abhay Kumar (2012), Aggregated Deflate-RLE compression technique for body sensor network." In *2012 CSI Sixth International Conference on Software Engineering (CONSEG)*, pp. 1–6. IEEE.

[17] Tiwari, V., & Tiwari, B. (2019). A Data Driven Multi-Layer Framework of Pervasive Information Computing System for eHealthcare. *International Journal of E-Health and Medical Communications (IJEHMC)* 10, no. 4 66–85.

[18] Ghamari, M., Janko, B., Sherratt, R. S., Harwin, W., Piechockic, R., & Soltanpur, C. (2016). A survey on wireless body area networks for ehealthcare systems in residential environments. *Sensors, 16*(6), 831.

[19] Tiwari, B. & Kumar, A. (2013). Physiological value based privacy preservation of patient's data using elliptic curve cryptography. *Health Informatics–An International Journal (HIIJ)* 2, no. 1 pp 1–14.

[20] Yadav, S., Tiwari, V., & Tiwari, B. (2016, March). Privacy preserving data mining with abridge time using vertical partition decision tree. In Proceedings of the ACM Symposium on Women in Research 2016 (pp. 158–164).

[21] Roempluk, T., & Surinta, O. (2019). A Machine Learning Approach for Detecting Distributed Denial of Service Attacks. In *2019 Joint International Conference on Digital Arts, Media and Technology with ECTI Northern Section Conference on Electrical, Electronics, Computer and Telecommunications Engineering (ECTI DAMT-NCON)* (pp. 146–149). IEEE..

[22] Garg, T., & Khurana, S. S. (2014, May). Comparison of classification techniques for intrusion detection dataset using WEKA. In *International conference on recent advances and innovations in engineering (ICRAIE-2014)* (pp. 1–5). IEEE..

[23] Bhattacharjee, P. S., Fujail, A. K. M., & Begum, S. A. (2017, December). A comparison of intrusion detection by K-means and fuzzy C-means clustering algorithm over the NSL-KDD dataset. In *2017 IEEE International Conference on Computational Intelligence and Computing Research (ICCIC)* (pp. 1–6). IEEE..

[24] Divyasree, T. H., & Sherly, K. K. (2018). A network intrusion detection system based on ensemble CVM using efficient feature selection approach. *Procedia computer science, 143*, 442–449.

[25] Aamir, M., & Zaidi, S. M. A. (2019). Clustering based semi-supervised machine learning for DDoS attack classification. *Journal of King Saud University-Computer and Information Sciences..*

[26] Vaseer, G., Ghai, G., & Patheja, P. S. (2017, December). A novel intrusion detection algorithm: An AODV routing protocol case study. In 2017 IEEE International Symposium on Nanoelectronic and Information Systems (iNIS) (pp. 111–116). IEEE.

[27] Batra, J. & Krishna, C. R. (2019). DDoS attack detection and prevention using Aodv routing mechanism and Ffbp neural network in a Manet. International Journal of Recent Technology and Engineering 8:2.

[28] Singh, N., Dumka, A., & Sharma, R. (2018) A novel technique to defend DDOS attack in manet. J Comput Eng Inf Technol 7:5.

[29] Intrusion Detection Evaluation Dataset (CIC-IDS2017). www.unb.ca/cic/datasets/ids-2017.html. 140

[30] Boukhamla, A., & Gaviro, J. C. (2021). CICIDS2017 dataset: performance improvements and validation as a robust intrusion detection system testbed. *International Journal of Information and Computer Security, 16*(1–2), 20–32.

[31] Kanimozhi, V., & Jacob, T. P. (2019, April). Artificial intelligence-based network intrusion detection with hyper-parameter optimization tuning on the realistic cyber dataset CSE-CIC-IDS2018 using cloud computing. In *2019 international conference on communication and signal processing (ICCSP)* (pp. 0033–0036). IEEE.

[32] Tavallaee, M., Bagheri, E., Lu, W., & Ghorbani, A. A. (2009, July). A detailed analysis of the KDD CUP 99 data set. In *2009 IEEE symposium on computational intelligence for security and defense applications* (pp. 1–6). IEEE.

Index